Warrior Fitness
Conditioning for Martial Arts

Jonathan Haas

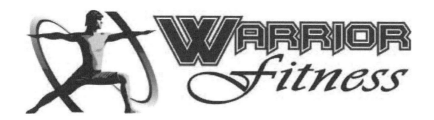

Medical Disclaimer

The material contained in this book is for informational purposes only. The author and all others affiliated with the creation, sale, and distribution of this book may NOT be held liable for any damages of any kind allegedly caused or resulting from any such claimed reliance. Before beginning this, or any, workout regimen, it recommended that you consult with your physician for clearance. The information contained herein is not intended to, and never should, substitute for qualified medical advice. If at any time you feel pain or discomfort, stop immediately.

Table of Contents

Medical Disclaimer 1

Dedication 5

Warrior's Creed 6

Forward 7

Introduction 8

    Supplementary Exercises or Just the Budo? 12

    What About Mixed Martial Arts? 14

Walking 15

Proprioception – the 6th Sense 18

    Proprioception Training 20

Flow Exercise 25

    Two Minute Flow Drill 28

Warrior Fitness 29

    Henka (Change/Vary) Your Exercises, but not too Often! 37

    Recovery and Restoration 39

    Joint Mobility Drills 41

    Flexibility 62

    Breathing 76

    Leg Training for Flexibility and Power 87

    The Core of a Warrior 96

    Upper Body Work 103

    Conditioning Exercises 114

Motivation 123

    How Often? 125

Creating a Training Program 127

    Strength Endurance Workout 128

    Explosive Strength Workout 129

    Conditioning for MA #1 129

    Conditioning for MA #2 (Minute Drills) 129

    Core Routine 130

    Warrior Fitness Sample Training Plan 131

Works Cited 133

About the Author 134

Dedication

This book is dedicated to my Grandfathers.

To my paternal grandfather, Peter Haas, Sr. (†) for introducing me to the idea of martial arts, and

To my maternal grandfather, Michael Minardi (†) for showing me what it truly means to be a warrior.

Warrior's Creed

By Robert L. Humphrey
(Iwo Jima Marine &
Bujinkan 10th Dan)

Wherever I go,
everyone is a little bit safer because I am there.
Wherever I am,
anyone in need has a friend.
Whenever I return home,
everyone is happy I am there.

"It's a better life!"

Forward

The great martial arts teacher, Masaaki Hatsumi said: "The first step in Ninpo training is that of physical endurance." Jon Haas' new book on Warrior Fitness is a welcome addition to any martial arts library. It weaves ancient admonitions on strength, flexibility and endurance with some of the latest fitness technology to assist sincere practitioners to attain a high level of physical efficacy.

I have known Jon since he walked into the training hall as a teenager. The road to true martial arts proficiency is long and hard. One can never assume that every person that starts down that path has the aptitude and persistence to "keep going." But Jon has not only walked the path with great consistency, he has balanced a heartfelt loyalty to his chosen martial tradition with an open and scientific mind. This book is a product of that unique synergy.

I heartily recommend that you read and study this book. I particularly recommend that you *use* it to increase and maintain a high level of fitness. Most of all, I challenge you to follow Jon's example and "keep going."

Jack Hoban

Introduction

The first two questions that come to my mind when I begin reading a book, especially on topics like health, fitness, or martial arts are:

1) Who is this person writing? And,
2) What are his qualifications?

Two very important questions when you are relying on the author for factual information, advice, and a qualified opinion.

What I have done is take an activity, martial arts, and make it a lifestyle. I have figured out, for myself, how to make this goal that we all have of continuous training (and continuous improvement) sustainable. In my eyes, physical fitness is an extremely important supplement to martial arts training. Because I view my health and fitness as a way to forge the complete "budo-body" necessary for continuous improvement in martial arts, I have spent considerable time and effort researching exercise science, reading the latest studies, and figuring out how to put that knowledge into practice for myself and my students. I am not a sports scientist. I do not possess a degree in exercise physiology. I do not work as a personal trainer. I am simply a martial artist. This is my story.

I began my odyssey into ninjutsu training years before my first actual formal instruction. It was the early 1980's and the "ninja boom" was in full swing. Since the only information I had to go on was based on Sho Kosugi movies, articles in Ninja magazine and some early Steven Hayes books, much of my training was creatively invented by me and some young, like-minded friends. Climbing trees, hiding in bushes, leaping and rolling over stumps, hedges, and throwing make believe shuriken at each other were just some of the things we did on a daily basis after school. I never knew it then, I just thought we were having fun, but those "ninja" games and fitness exercises we devised would serve me well as I began to explore Hatsumi Sensei's (Grandmaster of the Bujinkan Martial Arts) budo for real in the summer of 1989. I clearly remember sitting in the backseat of my parents' car reading the latest issue of Blackbelt Magazine when I came upon the full page advertisement for the 1989 Tai Kai (3 day training event) taught by Hatsumi Sensei. To my utter astonishment and immense excitement, I saw it was being held in Somerset, NJ, just 45 minutes from where I lived! A life changing moment occurred when I begged for my parent's permission to go (I was 16 at the time) and they agreed.

Shortly after a whirlwind 3 days of being exposed to Soke's budo with many of the Japanese, American, and European Shihan (master instructors), I quit the Okinawan Karate I had been practicing for years and began training under senior Bujinkan instructor, Jack Hoban. I trained with Jack as much as I could, usually 2 days a week and every monthly seminar, but still, it was not enough. I had an appetite for budo that 3 hours a week just could not satiate. How would I fill this hunger? Sensei's books were just becoming popular at that time, <u>Ninja Secrets from the Grandmaster</u>, <u>Essence of Ninjutsu</u>, etc. and I voraciously devoured them, but reading and thinking about training was still not enough.

"You learn to study by yourself... I often remind my students and myself, 'life is to practice by myself.'" (Hastumi, Ninpo: Wisdom for Life)

Many, many times in those early days (and still today!), Jack reminded us that the real training for budo was done at home. Classes and seminars are the fun part, he would say smiling, but the only way to achieve any type of progress is to train by yourself. Think about it. There are 168 hours in a week. If only 3 of them are spent training in a martial arts class, what are you doing for the other 165? Everything you do, or **don't do**, is an act of conditioning. If 165 hours a week are spent not doing anything related to training, then how much of an impact will those 3 hours of training really have on your overall development as a budoka? You will most likely have to spend every class relearning the same skills since your body cannot possibly assimilate them when trained only a couple times a week!

"Modern budo students often forget to practice by themselves. I used to practice by myself. When there was no teacher, I found the secret teachings by my own desire." (Hastumi, Ninpo: Wisdom for Life)

I took Jack's advice to heart and began devising my own budo training regimen that I would work on outside of class to supplement and augment the vast array of techniques and skills that I was learning from Jack and my sempai – seniors in the art. The early years, of course, were defined by trial and error where I would fail often more times than succeed. Luckily, I was too stubborn to give up and kept training and learning! This manual is the product of 17 years of research, thinking, planning, and training; in short, it is the manual I wish I had had back in 1989 when I first started training. Over the years I have been blessed to train with many wonderful Bujikan teachers, Jack Hoban, of course being primary, as well as some incredibly talented training partners who have become true Buyu (warrior friends).

Although much of the exploration for this manual, whether through research or practical application, took place by myself working in the laboratories of my basement, backyard, the woods, parks, my college dorm room, countless gyms, and hotel rooms while traveling for work, I would be extremely remiss if I did not also mention the students who have trained with me over the years while I refined my teaching ability and developed my training philosophy. They deserve a lot of credit for putting up with my constant dissatisfaction with ideas that could have been classified as "good enough" and for supplying me with indispensable feedback about which drills and exercises provided the most value for increasing performance in martial arts and which ones needed to be junked. This manual, of course, is comprised only of the most valuable.

Supplementary Exercises or Just the Budo?

"Considerable research and experience has shown that the system of using the sport alone to develop proficiency generally is less effective than the integrated system of sport and supplementary training." (Siff, Supertraining)

It is my contention, and the premise of this manual, that the above statement applies equally to martial art as it does to sports and athletics. Supplementary training for performance enhancement should go hand in hand with the traditional *budo keiko – martial arts practice*. If athletes at the uppermost echelons of their respective games can benefit from, and indeed, rely upon this type of training to carry their performance to the next level, why shouldn't we as *budoka* take advantage of the same ideas? These exercises are by no means an attempt to replace traditional skill acquisition in the martial arts, but are an effective way to supplement training and better prepare the body and mind for training. Rather, think of the exercises and drills presented in this manual as specific ways of priming the neurological pathways so that your body has a greater capacity to absorb the skills of Bujinkan Budo Taijutsu.

Functional exercise is defined as multi-planar, multi-joint movement, in other words, three dimensional movements. Since combat occurs in a volatile and unpredictable atmosphere, training must prepare the warrior to adapt. Remember that the goal of all the exercises in this manual is to develop the ability to control the degree of tension in our body and be able to utilize just the right amount of force at the appropriate moment. This way we may be able to sustain activity for longer and longer periods of time without exhausting our muscles. The example often given is that of a battle lasting several days. How did ancient warriors continue to function, no less fight, for that long a period of time? If they had used the principle of generalized tension throughout the entire body, the muscles would have burned out within the first few hours, long before the second or third day of combat! Strength training and muscular endurance training are a must, but the way in which they are trained is more important.

The program outlined in this book requires minimal equipment. All that is needed to create a Warrior Fit body is a pull-up bar (a tree branch or playground provide a handy substitute), a 4-foot long stick, your own body weight, and a little space!

What About Mixed Martial Arts?

Though the majority of the exercises in this manual may be applied to combat athletics, it is not really written with the intention of being a training guide for the "combat athlete." MMA, wrestling, and boxing are very different from warrior training and require specific (the way the exercises are trained is different – different training philosophy because they have divergent goals) strength and conditioning strategies separate from those contained herein. Although those sports require enormous physical skill and conditioning, the athletes that participate in them are usually only concerned with fighting a single opponent, in a symmetrical force-on-force engagement, trained in a similar manner with the same or similar skill set and in the same weight class. The bouts are timed and a referee is present to ensure no rules of the sporting engagement are broken and no one gets hurt (too much). Due to the concept of specificity in training, combat athletics and warrior arts by necessity require different training periodizations (schedules) and methodologies. The format for the drills and exercises presented here have been specifically researched and formulated for the physical and mental development for the student of the warrior arts, although with a change in their application and focus they may be adapted to combat athletics as well.

Walking

Proper walking is footwork training for budo. How we walk in day-to-day life is how we will walk (move) in combat. Efficiency in more complex movement begins with efficiency in simple movements. How can we expect to move with ease in the chaos of a combative environment when most of us have trouble walking with natural gait? Walking is a ubiquitous activity that many people simply take for granted. They move through the day without any awareness of the strain they place on their knees, hips, and lower backs by their poor movement patterns. Just a little awareness will do wonders for your balance, posture, and lightness of step. When Hatsumi Sensei first came to the U.S., of the things he noticed immediately was how heavy and inefficiently people walked. His comment was that most people walked "like Frankenstein"!

Walking exercises:

1. Stand in shizen no kamae (natural posture) and balance on one leg. Lift the other foot a few inches off the ground and then lower again in a slow, controlled manner using the flexing of the grounded leg to regulate the descent. Gently bounce a few times getting the feeling of how the grounded leg's flexion and extension controls the lowering of the other foot. The balance on your leg should be such that you are able to lower the opposite

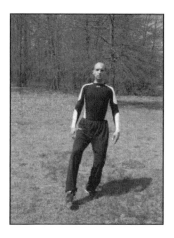

foot to the ground in any direction and easily maintain kamae (balance). Switch legs and now balance on the other leg while lowering the foot.

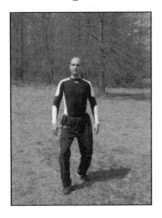 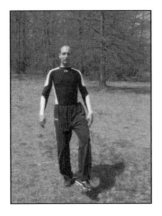 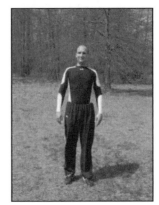

2. Stand in shizen no kamae (natural posture). Use your right hip to lift the right foot off the ground. It will feel strange at first since this is not a very commonly used muscle action, but once you get used to it, it will become an efficient way of lifting the leg. With the right leg lifted, pull back with the right shoulder.

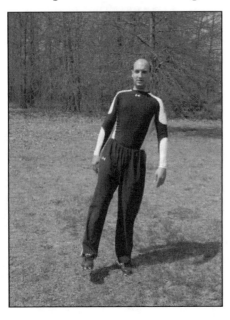 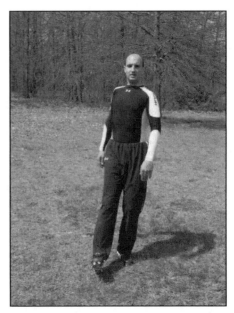

Notice how this has the effect of creating a slight torque in the spine and moves the right foot forward at the same time. Release the tension in the spine by placing the right foot down in a forward step. Feel how the release of tension propels the body forward and allow it to create the same lift from the hip and pulling back of the shoulder on the left side.

3. Combine the previous two exercises together and begin to walk.

Another idea to try when walking is to alternate periods of normal, regular breathing with holding your breath for duration when "full", after an inhale, and when "empty", after an exhale. Try inhaling for a count of 5 (steps or seconds), hold your breath for a count of 5, exhale for a count of 5, and finally, hold your breath empty for a count of 5 while walking. Repeat as long as you can continue the pace. Note that 5 is just an arbitrary number and can be raised or lowered to suit your own needs. This practice will help you to understand how your body can function during situations when you must suddenly hold your breath yet still continue to work. Another benefit of this exercise is that it also helps the body to process oxygen to brain, heart, and other working muscles more efficiently.

Don't forget "light feet and soft knees" when walking!

Proprioception – the 6th Sense

Science and Technology Encyclopedia defines "Proprioception" as:

> *The sense of position and movement of the limbs and the sense of muscular tension. The awareness of the orientation of the body in space and the direction, extent, and rate of movement of the limbs depend in part upon information derived from sensory receptors in the joints, tendons, and muscles. Information from these receptors, called proprioceptors, is normally integrated with that arising from vestibular receptors (which signal gravitational acceleration and changes in velocity of movements of the head), as well as from visual, auditory, and tactile receptors.*

Jack Hoban once described taijutsu as a dog fight between two jet fighters whirling around at crazy, unpredictable angles in three dimensional spaces as opposed to the two dimensional, head-to-head fights of battling tanks. In Jack's example, you can get an idea of how the development of this 6th Sense is extremely important in the context of budo training.

A simple test to determine the degree to which your body relies upon vision alone as its primary sense for balance and stability is to assume Ichimonji No Kamae (shown below), close your eyes, and then try to move into Hicho No Kamae (shown below).

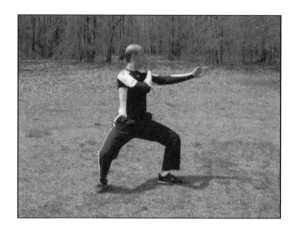
Ichimonji No Kamae

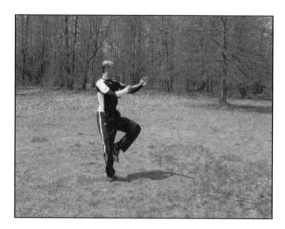
Hicho No Kamae

If you find yourself unable to do this successfully or are extremely wobbly, then your sense of proprioception is weak and underdeveloped. Continue to practice this simple exercise, but scan your body for unnecessary tensions. Feel the point(s) where you are slipping off balance and notice the misalignment in your structure (kamae) that is causing it. Train with awareness!

"One way of improving proprioceptive efficiency is to diminish or block input from other sensory systems such as the eyes…. Research has shown that blindfolding does not disrupt motor activities; on the contrary, it has been found that exercises are performed with greater precision and stability when the eyes are closed or in darkness. The athlete remembers joint angles; the degree of muscular tension, the amplitude of movement and movement patterns best with the eyes closed and reproduces them more easily. Subsequently, when the movements are done with the eyes open, the athlete's enhanced motor sensitivity is preserved and his technical skill improves." (Siff, Supertraining)

The degree of sophistication in this exercise can be increased by adding in more complex movements once you can successfully balance on your structure in Hicho no Kamae with eyes closed. The following are some examples:

Proprioception Training

The goal of these proprioception training exercises is to be able to move smoothly and efficiently, and to keep your balance easily whether your eyes are open or closed. The increased complexity of the exercises, combined with removing the sense of sight will aid in enhancing your body's proprioception.

1. Begin in left Hicho No Kamae (shown below), shift as smoothly as possible into right Hicho No Kamae (shown below).

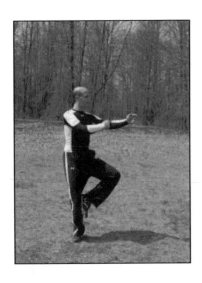
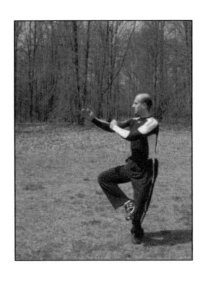

Left Hicho No Kamae   Right Hicho No Kamae

Keep your head in the same horizontal plane as you transition from left to right. Do these with your eyes open at first to "groove" the movement. Once you are comfortable, close your eyes and do it again. Suddenly it becomes difficult again, right?!

2. As above, begin in left Hicho No Kamae. This time, leap into right Hicho No Kamae. Keep your head in the same horizontal plane as you leap from left to right Hicho no kamae. Do these with your eyes open at first to "groove" the movement. Once you are comfortable, close your eyes and do it again.

3. Begin in left Hicho No Kamae, bend the right leg and lower the body as close as possible to the ground; perform a front roll into Ichimonji No Kamae. Do these with your eyes open at first to "groove" the movement.

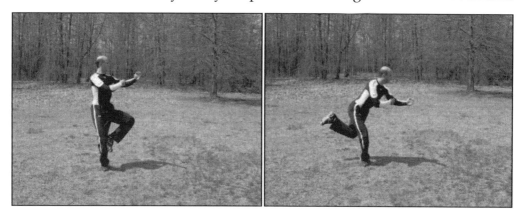

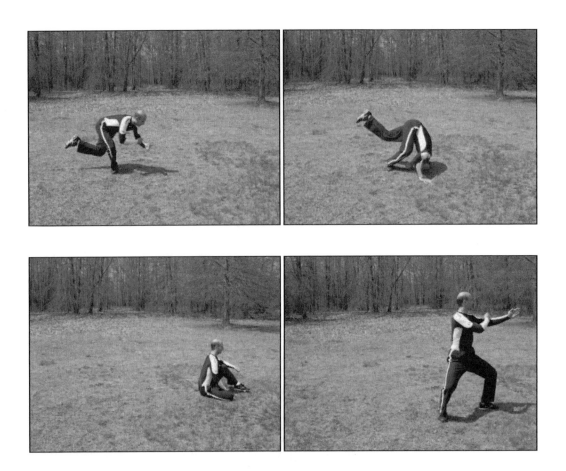

Once you are comfortable, close your eyes and do it again.

Now it's time to chain multiple movements together: Begin in left Ichimonji No Kamae. Move to Hicho No Kamae.

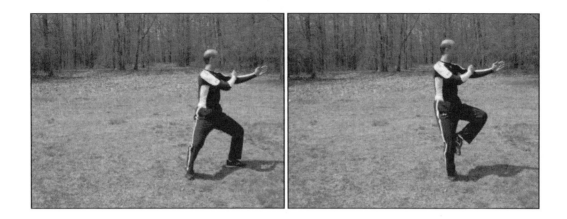

Cross step backward with your raised left leg into a right Ichimonji No Kamae.

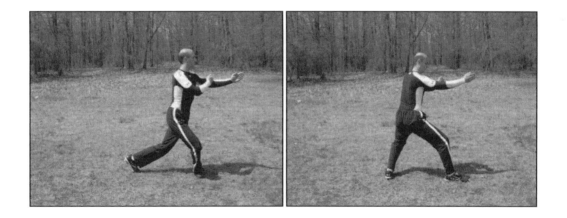

Pick the front leg up into Hicho no Kamae again, and front roll into right Ichimonji. Once you are comfortable, close your eyes and do it again.

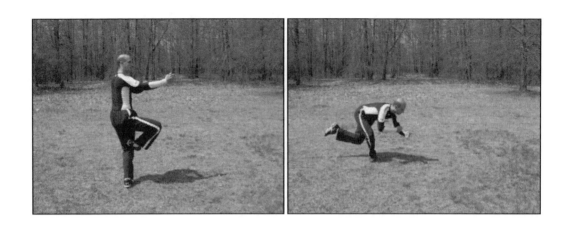

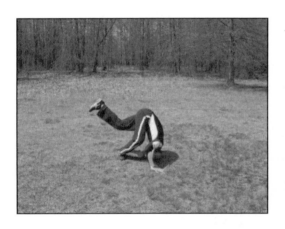
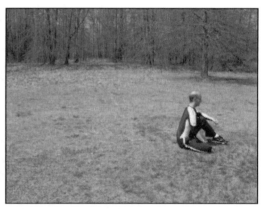

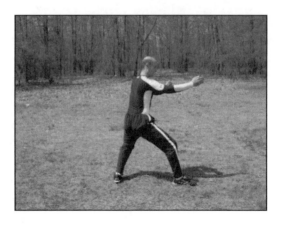

Flow Exercise

The next set of exercises is specifically designed to increase flow (nagare) in your taijutsu. However, before we get into the exercises themselves we should address the question, what is flow? Flow is efficiency and continuity in movement. Flow is smoothness of movement that is unencumbered by mechanical, jerky actions. Moving at a faster pace and working harder, does not necessarily mean that the movement is flowing. In fact, if you are working harder, I can almost guarantee the movement is not flowing. Flow is not something you do; it is something you get out of the way of! What types of internal distractions, tensions, hitches in movement are preventing you from getting out of your own way?

These flow exercises are culled from basic exercises of Bujinkan Budo Taijutsu, but can be utilized by anyone to expand your movement potential and increase flow. When training these exercises, the idea is, of course, continuous movement. Begin with a slow and smooth protocol, working on keeping a good technique level and efficient transition between the movements. One discovers the key to developing flow by examining the **in between stages of movement**. Often, we see the kamae (structure) and then we see the roll, but what we miss is the essence of flow – the small, transitory movements between them. Do not attempt to "accomplish" this exercise; that is not the point. Use it as a vehicle to unlock the flow in your movement. Try to keep moving. Don't pause to think in the middle. Increase the speed as you begin to feel comfortable, but if the technique begins to get sloppy or the movements begin to look mechanical, drop down the intensity level until you are once again performing the flows with good technique. Remember, there is zero training value in simply trying to do the exercises for a "cardio" workout. Go buy a treadmill!

1. Step back from a natural posture into left leg forward Ichimonji No Kamae. Do Chi No Kata. From the end point of the kata, continue lowering your center of gravity and extend the right arm to effectively blend the transition from Chi No Kata into a front roll. Allow the momentum of the front roll to carry you to your feet, lifting up from the crown of your head and using your spine, into right Ichimonji No Kamae and, without stopping in the kamae, leap forward landing again in right Ichimonji No Kamae. Continue the movement by reaching forward with the left hand with a feeling of the body being pulled by the hand into left Ichimonji No Kamae. Repeat on the other side.

2. Step back from a natural posture into left Ichimonji No Kamae. Do Sui No Kata. From the omote shutou strike at the end of the kata, continue lowering the body with the weight on the front leg, simultaneously stepping through with the back leg to transition from the strike into a back roll. Allow the momentum of the back roll to carry you to your feet, lifting up from the crown of your head and using your spine, into right Ichimonji No Kamae and, without stopping in the kamae, leap backward landing again in right Ichimonji No Kamae. Repeat on the other side.

3. Step back from a natural posture into left Ichimonji No Kamae. Do Ka No Kata. From the ura shutou strike at the end of the kata, bring your left foot forward next to the right foot a little more than shoulder width apart to transition into Hira No Kamae. Without stopping in the kamae, lower your center of gravity and flow into a side roll to the right. Roll right back into Hira No Kamae and leap sideways to the right, landing again in Hira No Kamae. Repeat on the other side.

4. Step back from a natural posture into left Ichimonji No Kamae. Do Fu No Kata. Immediately transition to Hoko No Kamae and flow into a cartwheel. Land back in Hoko No Kamae and leap down into a kneeling Ichimonji No Kamae. Repeat on the other side.

5. Step back from a natural posture into left Ichimonji No Kamae. Do Ku No Kata. Immediately transition to a forward breakfall followed by a forward roll into Jumonji No Kamae. Leap directly upwards. Repeat on the other side.

Two Minute Flow Drill

Use this drill to free yourself from constantly thinking about techniques. The goal of the drill is to perform any combination of strikes, kicks, ukemi (rolling), footwork, and taihenjutsu (body-changing art) without predetermining what you should do. Do not think. Do not stop. Keep going for the full 2 minutes. Continuous movement and flow between techniques is important. When you first start doing this exercise, you may find yourself repeating the same movements over and over again. That's fine. Keep going with it. Eventually you will begin to let go of your preconceived ideas and start to form true free-flowing movement. Make sure that every movement is done with an awareness of your kamae. Do not train bad habits!

Warrior Fitness

"Are you <u>FIT</u> to be a warrior?"

It goes without saying that the role of a warrior in the greater community is to protect yourself and others. Yet, how many of us aspiring warriors realize that health, fitness, and overall well-being are primary qualities that are on the forefront of "self" defense? Most of us may train our entire lives without ever being involved in a dangerous altercation, but the same cannot be said about avoiding the dangers of lack of physical exercise such as osteoarthritis, ill health, heart disease, cancer, type II diabetes, and obesity to name a few. Physical fitness (and proper nutrition!) plays a lead role in the prevention of these diseases and conditions, as well as in the protection of our overall health and psychological well being.

One area that appears to be lacking in the current training regimen of the majority of Bujinkan students is physical fitness and conditioning training. However, when we look back a few hundred years and compare the lifestyle of past practitioners to our current, modern lifestyle we begin to understand that they really didn't require a formalized fitness program because their normal daily activities kept them in good physical condition. It wasn't a necessary component of their training. Working in the fields was much more physically demanding than getting in a car and pushing a cart around the supermarket aisles. Unfortunately, our modern lifestyle has become extremely sedentary. We see the effects of this every day.

Most of us spend 40 + hours a week sitting in an office staring at a computer where the most exercise we get during an 8-hour stint is to walk to the bathroom several times a day followed by wandering into the cafeteria to see what pre-packaged garbage is waiting for us in the vending machines. Then, often we come home from work exhausted (from what?) and flop on the couch to watch TV in order to "unwind" (again, from what?) before finally dragging ourselves upstairs and into bed for the night. We have conditioned ourselves into laziness and inaction. Yes, I do mean "conditioned". Conditioning does not only apply to being fit; it is possible to condition your body for anything, including being overweight, tired all the time, and to completely lack motivation for any type of physical activity. No wonder Americans are among the fattest people on the planet! (By the way, I am only picking on Americans because I am one; however the rampant increase in obesity is a worldwide problem and getting worse. Just look at recent news articles from the UK on the same subject.)

One of the problems that arise when we attempt to discuss fitness is that the term itself is extraordinarily vague. Some people think of a tri-athlete as "fit" while others believe a power lifter is "fit." Unfortunately, neither of these examples conforms to the definition of fitness; they are just two ends of the spectrum. Fitness is actually made up of nine different components:

> Strength;
> Power;
> Agility;

- ➢ Balance;
- ➢ Flexibility;
- ➢ Local muscular endurance;
- ➢ Cardiovascular endurance;
- ➢ Strength endurance;
- ➢ Coordination

All of these components must be present to constitute a proper definition of fitness.

As martial artists we all generally tend to cringe and shy away from words like "strength" and "power" in favor of seemingly more budo-friendly words like "agility", "coordination", and "balance". Yet, often we do not understand the actual definitions of the words and simply avoid them because of some misplaced fear that they will be detrimental to our taijutsu and make us "muscle" through our techniques. Nothing could be further from the truth! Let's examine some of the components that make up fitness in more detail to understand just how much they are applicable to creating a strong physical and mental base from which to launch the rest of our budo taijutsu skills.

General physical conditioning is essential for the warrior to develop a broad-based platform of strength, endurance, agility, coordination, and flexibility from which to launch and further refine skills.

So, what exactly is strength? Strength is defined as "the ability of a given muscle or group of muscles to exert force against resistance." It is a function of the appropriate muscles contracted by effective nervous stimulation. This alone, however, is insufficient. There are also at least five different sub-categories of strength which we will break down to give you a more complete understanding of the term.

The first sub-category is **Maximal Strength**. This is the maximum amount of force that a person can voluntarily produce. Example exercises to cultivate Maximal Strength are: one arm pushups, one arm chin-ups, one legged squats, and heavy weight lifting. But what on earth does Maximal Strength have to do with Budo Taijutsu? Aren't we training to only use as much force as necessary and appropriate to a specific movement or technique? Why would we need our maximal voluntary strength output when training for taijutsu fitness? These are all good questions. On the surface, it would seem like this sub-category of strength is a big "N/A" for us. However, as martial artists, we are trained to look beyond the surface and research subjects deeply. Hatsumi Sensei is teaching a PhD program in Budo Taijutsu; we can't be content with a high school exercise science explanation. So, what possible benefit could this particular strength quality have for budoka?

To begin to appreciate the benefits of training maximal strength, we must first understand the different types of muscle fibers. Generally, when people speak about fast twitch and slow twitch muscle fibers, they tend to separate them out as two distinct types. This can be a little misleading due to the fact that muscle fibers are not either /or, but in actuality they appear to lie somewhere on a continuum between the two. Thus to emphatically state that one type or the other is predominate within certain groups of muscles can cause confusion.

Because low intensity exercise, like jogging at a steady-state pace for example, does not activate the fast twitch (FT) muscle fibers, we must increase the intensity of the exercise to stimulate the motor units that contain the FT fibers. If the motor units are not stimulated, then no response occurs and no adaptation occurs. Fast twitch muscle fibers and slow twitch muscle fibers are both recruited in high percentages when performing maximal strength exercises. Maximal strength training creates potent neural adaptations which lead to increased intermuscular and intramuscular coordination. A side bonus for working on maximal strength with body weight exercises is that the majority of them that fall in this category also require balance, coordination, flexibility, and appropriate tension throughout the entire body. Examples include, but are by no means limited to, one arm push-ups, one-legged squats, one arm chin-ups/pull-ups, etc.

Does this mean that we should devote every training session to developing maximal strength? No – far from! As warriors, we must understand the different qualities that make up strength and learn how to apply them to optimize our fitness levels specific to our goals. Since our goals do not revolve around winning any Strongman competitions or Power lifting contests, we can relegate working on maximal strength to only once a week, at the most, or a every couple weeks at the very least, to reap the benefits. The rest of the time, consign maximal strength to its rightful place back in our strength and conditioning toolbox. Too much emphasis on maximal strength can lead to becoming muscle "bound", as in bound, constrained, unable to move freely and without appropriate tension.

The second sub-category of Strength is **Explosive Strength**. This is the ability to produce maximal force (see above) in a minimal amount of time. Explosive strength? Jon, you've got to be kidding me! We don't use explosive strength in Bujinkan Budo Taijutsu! Really? Are you sure? Every time you leap, sprint, dive out of the way of an errant sword strike, or (and this is a big one!) use stored elastic energy to create power in your movement, you are using explosive strength. Sure, the terminology sounds like something that will adversely affect our taijutsu and that any serious budoka should avoid like the plague, but rest assured, that the much maligned concept of strength does play an important role in budo taijutsu and utilizing the strength exercises prescribed in this manual will provide a solid physical basis on which to build real skill.

Plyometrics is a specific training means for developing explosive strength designed by Russian sports scientist, Yuri Verkhoshansky in the early 1960's. We will examine several different plyometric exercises later in the text.

Closely linked to Explosive Strength are Speed Strength and Reactive Strength.

The third sub-category of strength is probably one of the most familiar to us. It is **Strength-Endurance**. Ok; much better… now we are in familiar territory. Endurance is a concept that a ninja can relate to! This strength quality involves the production of muscular tension without a noticeable decrease in efficiency over long periods of time. Development of strength-endurance is a fundamental necessity for warriors, whether on the battlefield, in training, or just everyday life.

A helpful analogy to keep in mind when applying the different aspects of strength training to budo is a recipe. All of the ingredients in any recipe are not utilized in the same amounts. A little bit of salt may be all that's required to enhance the flavor, while a lot of flour may be necessary to provide the base. The same idea applies to strength training. Warriors will normally require a lot of strength endurance and cardio-respitory endurance, but maybe only a little bit of maximal strength development is necessary to round out their overall skill.

"When effective methodology is used, exercises with resistance promote not only an increase in movement speed but also perfection of coordination, motor reaction, quickness and frequency of movements, the ability to relax muscles, development of local muscular endurance and an increase in maximal anaerobic capacity." (Verkhoshansky, Special Strength Training – A Practical Manual for Coaches)

The key here is in how these various strength qualities are trained. For martial arts, specifically Bujinkan Budo Taijutsu, we want to work exercises which emphasize intermuscular coordination of the whole body. Isolation exercises should be avoided as they are antithetical to what we are trying to accomplish in training. When performing all of the exercises listed here, try to use as little tension and muscular effort as possible; just enough to accomplish the task and no more. Try not to utilize general tension (tightening of the entire body) to carry you through the exercise. Since everything that we do acts as conditioning for our Central Nervous System (CNS), for good or for bad, we want to make sure our exercise philosophy is in harmony with our overall training strategy. Remember that in our day-to-day Bujinkan Budo training we are striving to perform techniques efficiently and effectively with minimal muscular recruitment, therefore our physical fitness training should not use a separate strategy.

The other important tip to remember in regards to fitness exercises is that most, if not all, the exercises performed should integrate the whole body. Isolation exercises should be left to the body-building crowd. Not that there's anything wrong with body-building as a sport; it's just not what we are training for.

In training, we are often admonished to "relax" and to move without using any tension. This, unfortunately, is impossible. We are physiologically unable to move without using tension – our bodies would crumple to the ground in a heap if we were truly without tension. A better way to phrase this idea is to "move with appropriate tension." This means using just enough tension, force, effort, muscle, to accomplish the movement and no more. It is important to note that both tension and relaxation are needed in training; they are two sides of the same coin. One cannot exist without the other. There is no such thing as being "completely relaxed"; the only way to be completely relaxed is to be dead.

Henka (Change/Vary) Your Exercises, but not too Often!

In order for the body to produce an adaptation for improved performance in life, sport, or budo, we must apply specific stimulus as per the SAID Principle (Specific Adaptation to Imposed Demand). This basically means that the body adapts with a specific type of fitness to any demand which is imposed on it. When the same exercise is performed for too long, the body adapts to the stresses of each set and the adaptations or returns get smaller and smaller. Once it has adapted to the stress, then it's time to change or increase the stress or else we fall into that trap of diminishing returns. The other thing that tends to happen when carrying out a particular exercise for longer than the period of adaptation is that boredom sets in! The exercise not only begins to loose its benefit to your training regimen, but it becomes monotonous and dull as well!

Usually after a period of 4-to-6 weeks it is a good practice to begin changing exercises. This does not mean that we need to completely throw away everything we have been doing; far from it. An exercise or drill can be changed by increasing intensity, increasing volume, decreasing rest periods, or increasing complexity or sophistication. Just like techniques within in taijutsu, there are many ways and variations in exercise routines. A corollary to this idea of changing exercises every 4-to-6 weeks is that some exercises in this book may take you much longer to even begin to do properly. Before setting about to change your routine, routinely, understand that some things require a lot more practice and effort before they can be simply plugged in and pulled out of your practice session.

A common principle within athletics is the idea of *overloading*. This principle states that "performance will increase only if athletes work at their maximum capacity against workloads that are higher than they encounter normally." In other words, the training load keeps increasing exponentially and this is supposed to correspond to an increase in strength/performance. The problem with this principle is that it was developed in a laboratory, in a vacuum, without the benefit of real world experience and vetting. This type of training over a long period of time will eventually result in overtraining, burnout, and injury. It is not possible to forever keep increase training loads and expecting the body to adapt. A better way to train is to realize that the body requires periods of rest and recovery as well as sub-maximal training loads interspersed with bouts of high intensity training in order to adapt and continue to improve performance over time.

Remember the saying – henka is the spice of life!

Recovery and Restoration

Intense training is necessary to push the envelope and truly begin to understand just how incredible this thing is that we call the human body. It is capable of many amazing feats and can be extraordinarily resilient, as long as we take proper care of it. Proper care includes knowing when to push further and when to allow the body time to relax. Without recovery and restoration periods interspersed throughout our training program, we would never be able to keep up continuous improvement (see the reference in the previous section to the principle of overloading). Constant, intense training by itself will invariably lead to overtraining, sickness, and injury. This is obviously not consistent with our overall warrior philosophy.

Unless you are overtraining, you should not have to take a complete rest day, no exercise at all, on a weekly basis. By planning your active recovery days into your weekly workout sessions and alternating the intensity of the workouts, your body should be able to adapt to the stress of the exercise and keep improving. If you find that you are feeling over tired, burnt out, or sick, you should obviously use your best judgment and take a day off. The number of complete rest days taken during the training week is obviously up to the individual. Normally, I take 1 to 2 full rest days in between each cycle (4 to 6 weeks) to allow my body to regenerate, recover, and assimilate the skills I have been working on in my training sessions. Depending on your level of overall conditioning, you may require one, two, or even three days of passive recovery – complete rest. The best way to determine how many rest days to program into your schedule is to experiment with it. If you are new to working out regularly then your body will require more rest than someone who has a solid general physical preparedness base.

Methods of Active Recovery:

➢ Joint mobility and stretching, both dynamic and static (discussed next chapter)

➢ Light jogging

➢ Massage

➢ Breathing exercises to re-oxygenate the blood (discussed later)

➢ Contrast bathing - This method involves the use of hot and cold water to alternatively dilate and then constrict blood flow to muscles. This acts to flush toxins out of the muscles and infuse them with "new" blood. In your post-exercise shower, begin with hot water, as hot as you can take it, for 40 seconds, then switch to cold water, as cold as you can take it, for 20 seconds. Repeat 4 to 5 times.

Joint Mobility Drills

Joint mobility is essential for lubricating the joints, loosening up the body, and increasing blood flow to aid in warming-up and injury prevention. Pain, stress, and tension are stored at various points in our bodies and can be abated and released through specifically designed mobility exercises. These exercise work by providing nutrition to the joints through synovial fluid and by breaking up deposits of sediment that can build up and "rust" our joints. Mobility training also works to increase the range of motion in our joints, muscles and connective tissues. By training yourself to be able to move slightly outside your comfort zone you are building in a safety-valve for when things happen to go wrong.

Also, there may be areas in the body where you may be storing tension that are detrimental to your performance since they are sapping energy and you are unaware of them. This is the basis for using dynamic mobility drills and active stretching (as opposed to passive) to release unnecessary tension to allow fuller, more powerful movement throughout an increased range of motion.

"For the competitive athlete or rehabilitative patient, static stretching is insufficient to develop the full range of movement strength, power, mobility and stability required in sport (or martial art)" (Siff, Supertraining)

The best time to do these drills is first thing in the morning. They serve as an early morning recharge for the entire body which will set the tone for the entire day. They can also be used prior to training or working out as a warm-up as well as after a workout, or between sets, to remove residual tension.

Try waking up 20 minutes earlier than usual and performing the following set of exercises. We'll begin with the neck and work our way down the body, covering all the joints.

Neck

1. Up/Down - lift up from crown of head; slide down along plane of jaw for 3 to 6 repetitions.

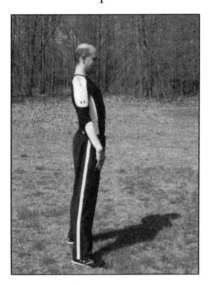 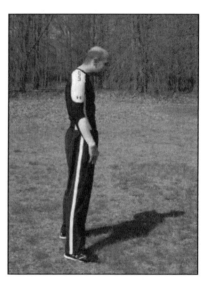

2. Left/Right - turn head as far left as possible without pain, turn as far right as possible for 3 to 6 repetitions.

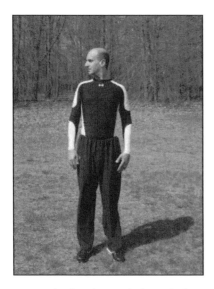 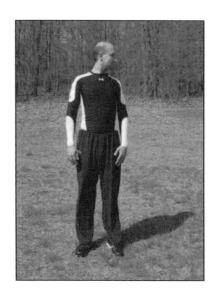

3. Side/Side - tilt head down to left; lift up from corner of jaw, repeat to right for 3 to 6 repetitions.

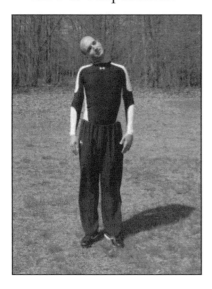 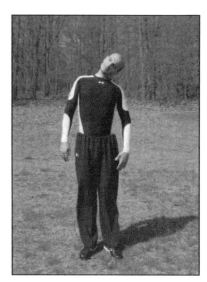

4. Full circles – both directions.

Shoulders

1. Roll both shoulders - lift shoulders up towards ears, roll backward fully articulating the range of motion (ROM), drop them down as far as comfortable for 3 repetitions, then repeat by rolling forward for 3 reps.
2. Alternate shoulder rolls - roll left shoulder back as described above while pushing right shoulder forward then switch. Perform 3 times each.

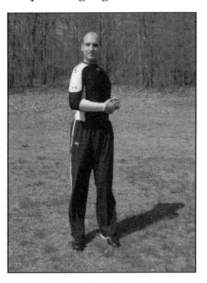 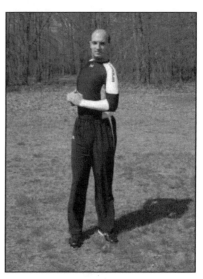

Arm Swings

1. Left to right - Begin with the right arm. Keep it naturally straight and swing in a figure 8 from left to right for 3 to 6 repetitions.

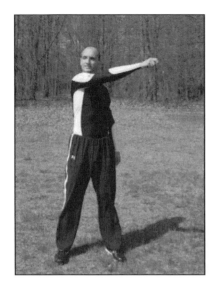 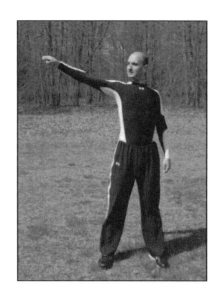

2. Reverse the direction and swing from right to left. Switch arms and repeat.

3. Bottom to top - Begin with the right arm. Keep it naturally straight and swing in a figure 8 from bottom to top.

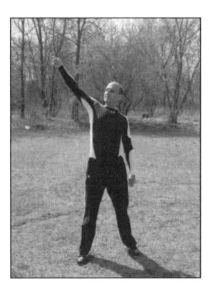 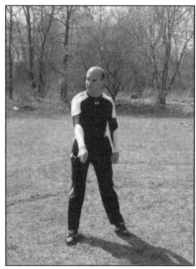

4. Front to back - Begin with the right arm. Keep it naturally straight and swing in a figure 8 from front to back.

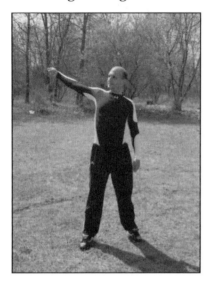
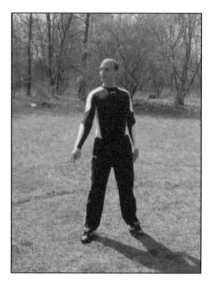
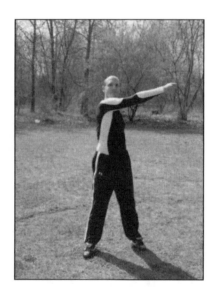

Elbows

1. Left/Right - rotate elbows in a left to right figure 8 for 3 reps. Switch directions.

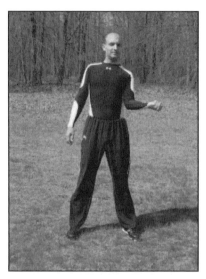
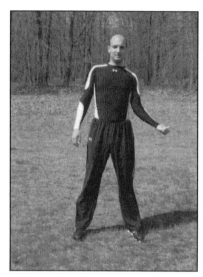
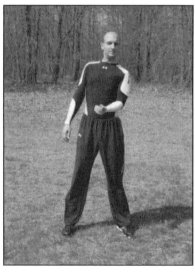
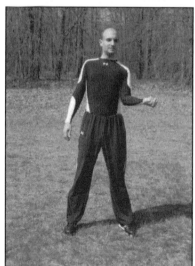

2. Top/Bottom - rotate elbow top to bottom in a vertical figure 8 for 3 reps. Switch directions.

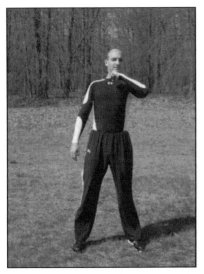
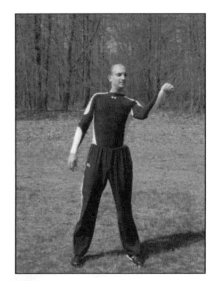
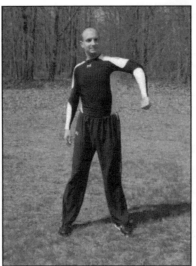

Wrists

1. Hold both hands in loose fists, make circles clockwise and counter clockwise with wrists. 3 reps in each direction.

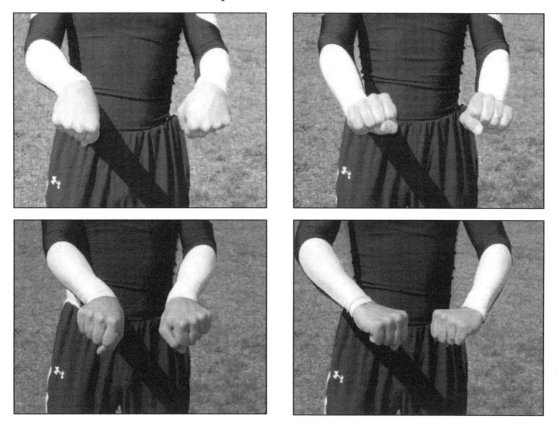

2. Begin with left wrist, hold in fist as above, lift wrist up, to the outside, down, to the inside, reverse direction and repeat with right wrist.

Fingers

1. Begin circling fingers with thumb 5 times, and then continue with each additional finger.

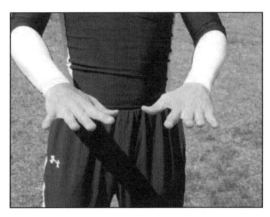

2. Circle fingers from pinky to thumb in the opposite direction

Chest

1. Without moving your pelvis, slide your thoracic cavity, left to right 3 times each direction.

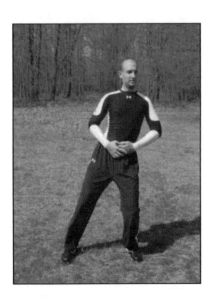 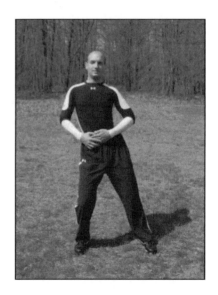

2. Forward/backward – inhale as you lift the chest up at a 45 degree angle, and then exhale as you move backwards. 3 times each.

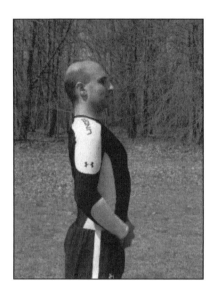 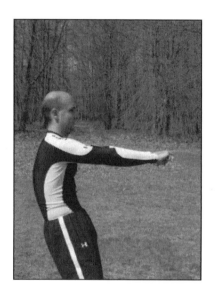

3. Make full circles with your chest: left, right, front, back, then reverse direction.

Hips/Pelvis

1. Circle hips clockwise and counter-clockwise 3 times in each direction.

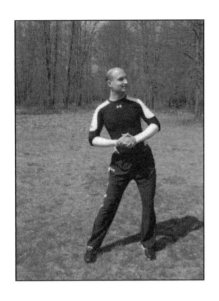
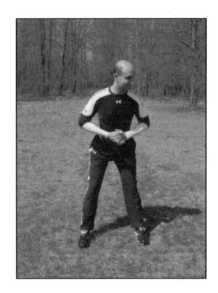
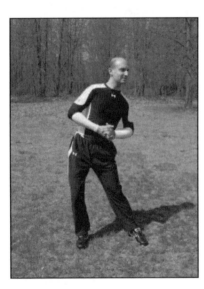
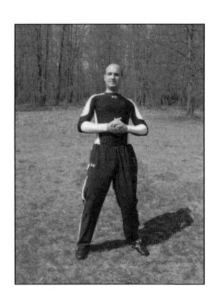

2. Tilt pelvis forward, backward, left, and then right.

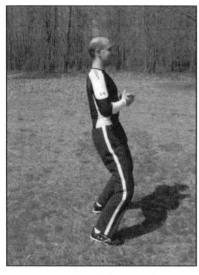
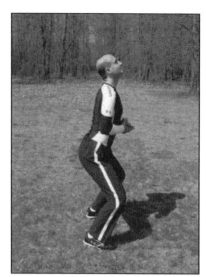
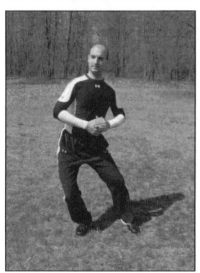
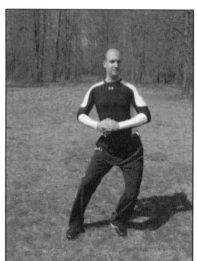

3. Put all 4 pelvic tilts into a continuous flow.
4. Use the hip to lift the leg straight upwards.

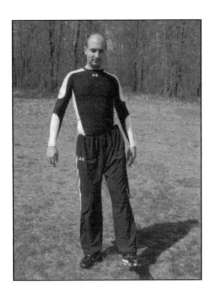 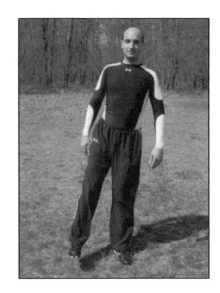

Spine

1. Keep the spine straight and fold forward at the hips, then rotate around to the left and back to center, then forward and around to the right.

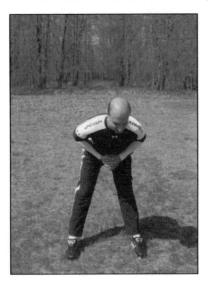 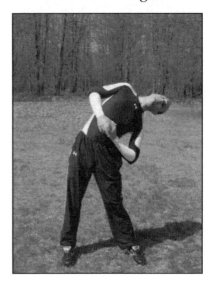

2. Keep the spine straight and fold backward at the hips, then rotate around to the left and back to center, then forward and around to the right.

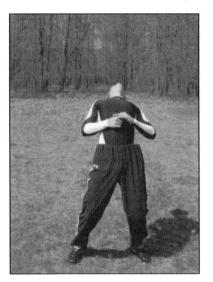 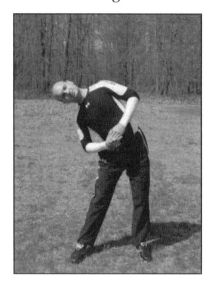

Knees

1. Massage both knee caps in a circular manner – both directions.

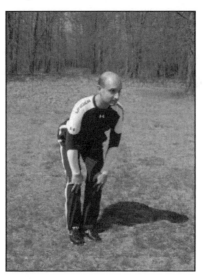

2. Palm knee caps and rotate knees to the left and to the right 3 to 5 times.

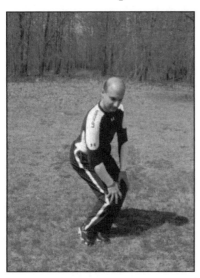
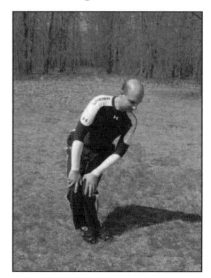

3. Lift one leg up in front so the thigh is parallel to the ground. Extend the lower leg to approximately a 45 degree angle and rotate the lower leg in both directions.

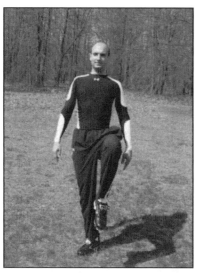
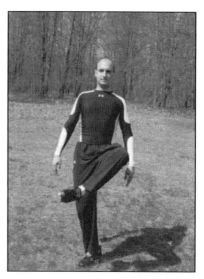
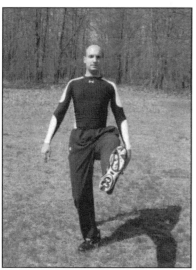
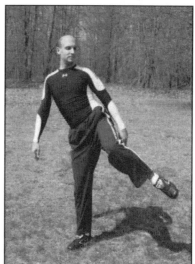

4. Repeat with the other leg.

5. Lift one leg up to the side. Extend the lower leg to approximately a 45 degree

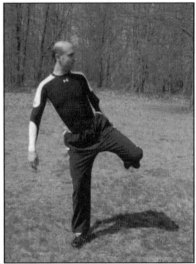

angle and rotate the lower leg in both directions.

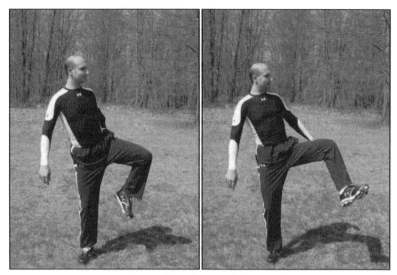
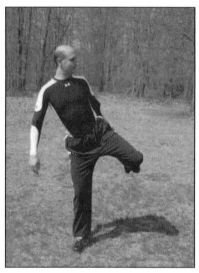

Ankles

1. Stand on one leg holding the other about 6 inches off the ground.

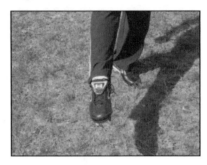

2. Extend the foot forward as far as possible, then flex back as far as possible. Do this 3 to 5 times each.

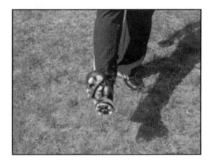

3. Next, turn ankle inwards towards centerline, then outwards 3-5 times.

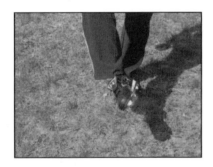
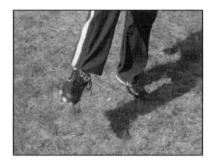

4. Now put all of them together and circle the joint in both directions 3-5 times each. Switch legs.

Leg Swings

1. Balance on one leg and begin to slowly swing the leg back and forth. As you become comfortable, begin to swing the leg higher and higher. Repeat 10 times per leg.

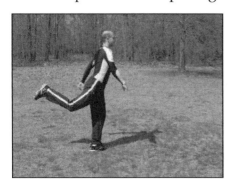 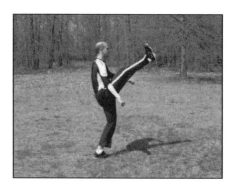

Flexibility

"The study of budo begins with giving flexibility to the legs and hips making them strong and supple."(Hatsumi, Togakure Ryu Ninpo Taijutsu)

Flexibility and range of motion in the hips and legs is essential for being able to move smoothly within kamae and transition efficiently between kamae, as well as for ukemi and taihenjutsu. The stretching exercises shown here will be dynamic flexibility ones where we are moving through and expanding a range of motion necessary for budo taijutsu. Dynamic flexibility exercises are useful for warming up prior to training or waking up first thing in the morning, while static flexibility exercises are more beneficial for a cool down, post-workout or relaxing before bed.

Ichimonji Leg Stretch

1. Bend front knee as far forward as possible while keeping the spine straight.

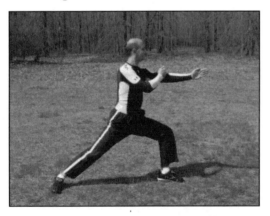

2. Allow back leg to straighten at the fullest extension of the stretch.

3. Rock hips/pelvis back and forth gently to loosen a little more and increase range of motion (ROM).
4. Back to center.
5. Rotate hips/pelvis circularly in both directions to increase ROM.
6. Reverse stretch by now bending back leg as far as possible while maintaining foot, hip, spine alignment.

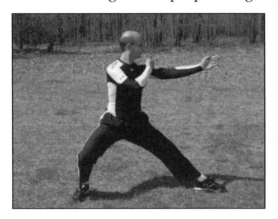

7. Allow front leg to straighten at the fullest extension of the stretch.
8. Rock hips/pelvis back and forth gently to loosen a little more and increase ROM.
9. Back to center.

Hira Leg Stretch
1. Bend right knee as far as possible while maintaining Hira No Kamae alignment.
2. Allow the left leg to straighten at the fullest extension of the stretch.
3. Rock hips/pelvis back and forth gently to loosen a little more and increase ROM.

4. Back to center.
5. Rotate hips/pelvis circularly in both directions to increase ROM,
6. Reverse stretch by now bending the left leg as far as possible while maintaining foot, hip, spine alignment,
7. Allow right leg to straighten at the fullest extension of the stretch,
8. Rock hips/pelvis back and forth gently to loosen a little more and increase ROM.

Squat Stretch
1. Turn both feet out at 90 degree angles.
2. Squat down as far as possible while still retaining an erect spine.

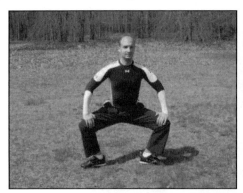
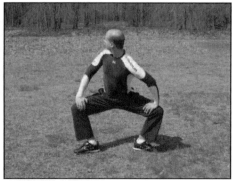
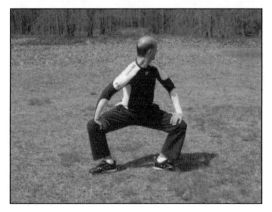

3. Place both hands on the knees and transfer your weight from side to side to begin loosening the hips.

Warrior Flexibility Series

1. Begin from Ichimonji no kamae stretch down to ground.

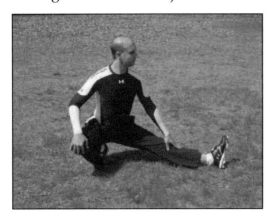 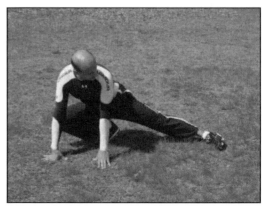

2. Rotate the extended leg to inside.

3. Continue rotating around from a mountain climber position into seated

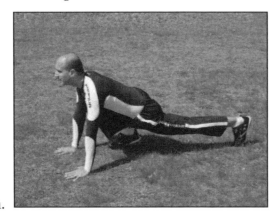

position.

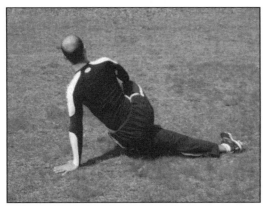

4. Release the torque and rotate back through previous positions into Ichimonji No Kamae again.
5. Switch into opposite Ichimonji No Kamae and repeat in the opposite direction.
6. From a Downward Facing Dog posture, push hips back to stretch spine.

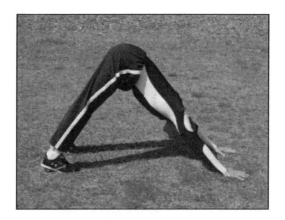

7. Exhale and reach your left hand to your right foot. Inhale as you come back to Downward Facing Dog. Exhale again and reach your right hand to your left foot.

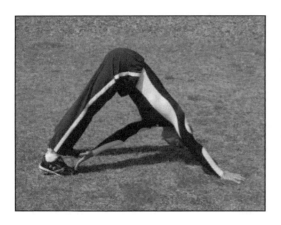 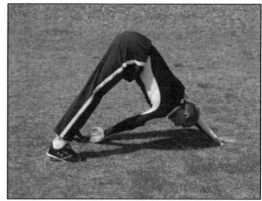

8. Move into Upward Facing Dog. Look over both shoulders to stretch spine to both sides.

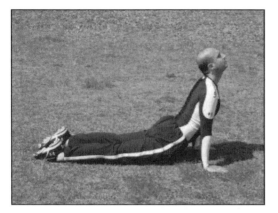
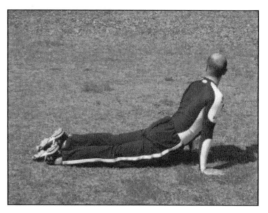
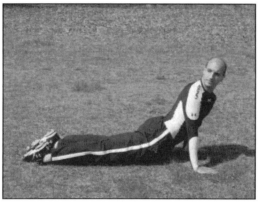

9. From Upward Facing Dog, push the hips back into seiza (kneeling posture) while keeping hands on ground to stretch spine. Move back and forth 4 to 5 times between these postures.

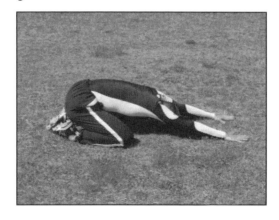

Yoga Compensatory Movement Routine

Traditional yoga teaches that balance in all things is very important to being a complete, healthy human being. This is accomplished through a process of compensatory movements designed to regulate and balance the entire human system so that no one area is overloaded. For example, after working through a series on backbends, the yoga routine will bring the practitioner's body back to a neutral position by including a forward bend. In Warrior Fitness, we take this concept and extrapolate it out to apply to a wider selection of exercises and physical movements. This ensures that our training, while intense, will not injure our bodies, but instead allow us to grow and continue to push the limits of our physical training no matter what our age.

This routine is designed to stretch out your entire body, but will focus on specific areas of tension like shoulders, hips, and hamstrings.

1. Begin in Child's Pose, arms stretched out straight in front to lengthen spine.

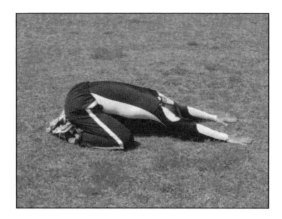
Child's Pose

2. Move into Upward Facing Dog, shoulders packed & down, chest expanded, head tilted up and back.

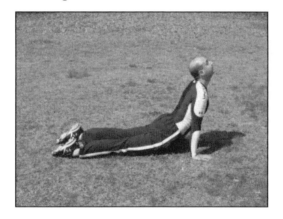
Upward Facing Dog

3. Back to Child's Pose, stretch deeper.

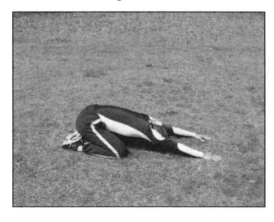

4. Back to Upward Facing Dog. Repeat one more time.
5. Move from Upward Facing Dog to Downward Facing Dog.

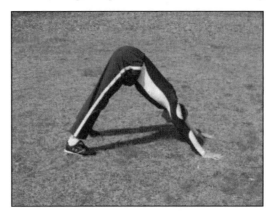

Downward Facing Dog

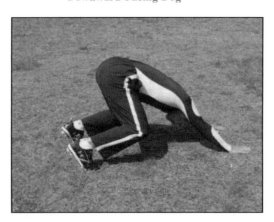

6. Drop knees to level of heels (don't let them touch the floor), tilt pelvis back towards your head, extend back to Downward Facing Dog.

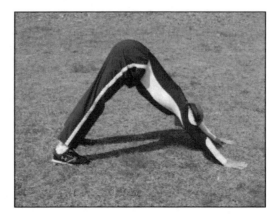

7. Drop knees to floor - Camel Pose. Move into and out of Camel Pose 4 times with breathing, then hold for 5 breaths.

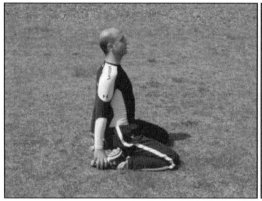 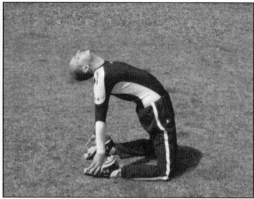

Camel Pose

8. Lie on your back and do a Shoulder Bridge. Move into and out of the Shoulder Bridge 4 times with breath before holding for 5 breaths.

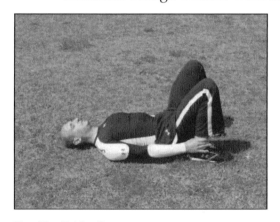 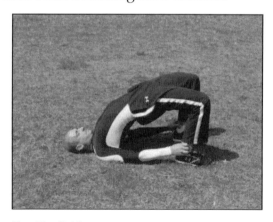

Shoulder Bridge Prep   Shoulder Bridge

9. Reach legs behind head for Plow Pose. Exhale, stretch deeper.

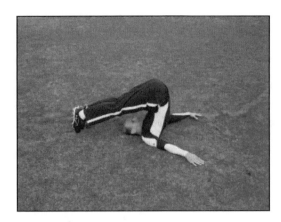

Plow Pose

10. Rock forward, stretch legs straight out in front, exhale and grab feet (or as close as possible). Inhale, come up. Exhale, back down. Repeat 2 more times, then hold for 5 breaths.

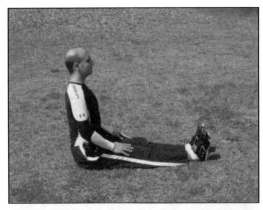

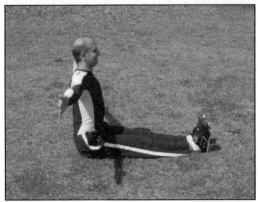

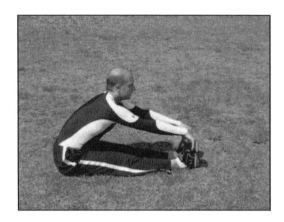

11. Sit up and then lie all the way back into Corpse Pose. Relax.

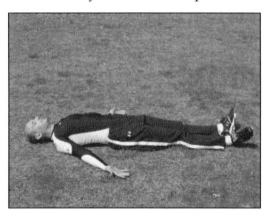

Breathing

"Breathing is natural." This is the typical response received when asking about breathing exercises in the Bujinkan. This statement is true, to an extent. Walking is probably one of the most natural things in the world for a bipedal human animal, yet how many of us study how to walk in depth (including in this manual!) in order to make it more "natural"? But when it comes to breathing, this topic is glossed over and we are simply told not to worry about it since breath should just be natural. Since breathing, by default, is far more important to our continued survival (past five minutes or so) than walking, shouldn't we at least investigate the topic, research and study it and practice it so that it becomes natural? Breathing obstructions can cause unconscious tension, tightness, lack of flexibility, and interfere with smooth, efficient movement. Unconscious holding of the breath during stressful situations can cause us to panic by increasing heart rate, blood pressure, and hinder us from being able to access our "natural" response. Poor conditioning can result in us being chronically "out of breath" during training or even something as simple as climbing stairs. The reverse is also true. Correct breathing can be used to calm you down in a stressful situation by lowering your heart rate and blood pressure. It can be used to boost energy when feeling tired or to relax and help you sleep. Fluid, deep breathing also serves to invigorate and energize every cell in our body, flushing them with healing energy and removing waste products. Another important fact to remember when attempting to understand the value of breathing exercises and why we should learn to control our breath is that breathing is the only bodily function that is both autonomic and voluntary. Because of this, there is enormous potential for using breathing to influence other bodily systems that we do not have conscious control over, such as your heart rate. This section will delve into the question of how we train our breath within the greater context of Bujinkan Budo Taijutsu.

Because the topic of breathing exercises has fascinated me for years, I have committed a vast amount of time to reading, researching, and practicing various breathing methods ranging from Chinese Qigong and Indian Yoga to the breathing practices taught in the Russian Martial Arts of ROSS and Systema. There is literally a ton of material available on ancient and modern breath training practices due to the recent openness and willingness of long time practitioners of various disciplines and sports scientists to share information. Cultural differences, archaic practices, and mythological references tend to obscure them on the surface making some things like yoga and qigong appear impenetrable without years of direct study under a qualified master of the arts. One of the most significant conclusions that I have drawn after years of examining these diverse systems is that once the principles and the physiology behind them are understood, the systems themselves become much easier to comprehend.

Some general principles that I have pulled from the various resources listed above and applied through practical experience are (in no particular order):

- Breathe in through the nose and out through the mouth

- Breathing should be constant with natural pauses between breath cycles, no unconscious holding of the breath (unless specifically working on a breath holding exercise)
- Breathing should not be fanatical – don't get caught in the trap of trying to match a particular phase of the breath cycle to a particular action, i.e., always trying to exhale when you punch or something equally silly.
- A corollary to the above principle though is that certain actions will naturally favor an inhale or an exhale. In those cases, then yes, follow the path of least resistance. Normally when the body contracts air is expelled from the lungs by the movement; allow it to happen. When the body expands, air is naturally sucked into the lungs; allow it to happen.
- Don't try to force yourself to breathe – allow it to happen (see above)
- Keep your spine straight, i.e. good posture, good kamae, is essential for unimpeded breathing

Although most systems of breath work are compatible with budo taijutsu, some, such as power breathing for example, generally may be contraindicated. The reason for this statement is due to the fact that usage of power breathing requires a high state of general tension throughout the entire body combined with extreme intra-abdominal pressure which is used to brace and stabilize the spine when lifting heavy loads. These characteristics of power breathing make it a poor choice for the Bujinkan practitioner due to the SAID principle. We do not want to create an adaptation in our organism that causes us to become rigid and hold our breath anytime we encounter resistance. Fluid, efficient movement using appropriate tension is our goal!

"Breathing is evidence of a living human being, and it is vital to grasp correct breathing that is truly in accord with the natural rhythm. In training, it is breath that gives life to and actualizes the technique(s)." (Hatsumi, Togakure Ninpo Taijutsu)

A great breathing exercise to practice first thing in the morning, or whenever you feel your energy levels sagging, to wake you up and get your body ramped up for the day is from yoga, called Kapalabahati (Skull Brightener). Kapalabahati is comprised of short, rapid exhalations, followed by short, rapid inhalations. The abdomen is quickly contracted on the exhale and released on the inhale in order to "pulse" the breath. Traditionally both are performed through the nose, but it may be easier for a person not used to this practice to exhale through the mouth. Generally, it is easier to modulate the volume of air exhaled through the mouth than through the nose, at least until you develop some degree of comfort with the practice.

On the other end of the spectrum, in order to lower your heart rate, blood pressure, and calm yourself down when overly nervous or anxious, the breath should be lengthened. Research has shown that tension increases slightly in the body during inhalation and lowers during exhalation. This practice of lengthening the exhalation can be used to a greater degree by keeping your inhalation relatively short, say 4-5 seconds, while stretching your exhalation out to 8-10 seconds. Continue this practice for about 10 full breaths to relax and calm yourself down.

Bujinkan Breathing Exercises

(Adapted from Hatsumi Sensei's Togakure Ninpo Taijutsu book)

Shomen Kokyuhou (frontal breathing)

1. Sit in seiza.

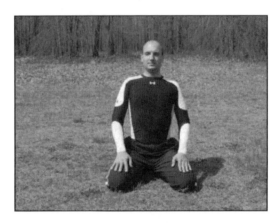

2. Open the shoulders and chest to allow a deep inhalation.

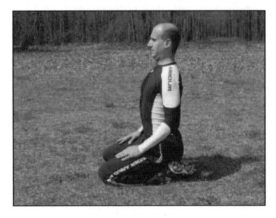

3. Drop shoulders to cause a compression of lungs and breathe out completely.

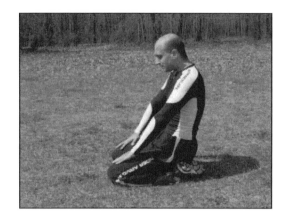

4. Repeat 8 times.

Seiza Sayuu Shinkokyuu (sitting left and right breathing)

1. Sit in seiza.

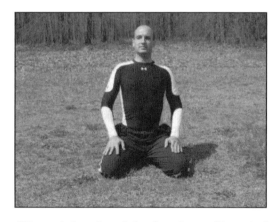

2. Turn to the right, pulling right shoulder back to allow inhalation.

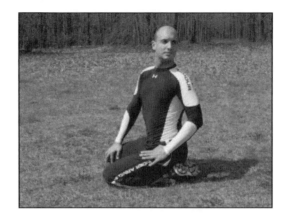

3. Release right shoulder and turn back to front allowing a complete exhalation. Repeat 8 times.
4. Repeat to the left side.

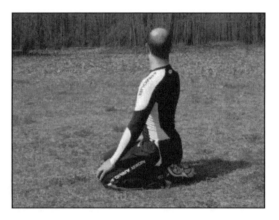

Shinten Shinkokyuu (extension deep breathing)

1. Sit with legs extended straight out in front of you.

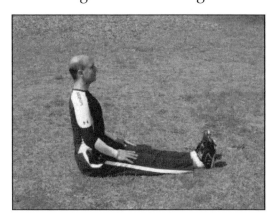

2. Open your arms wide out to the sides. Raise arms above your head as you inhale deeply.

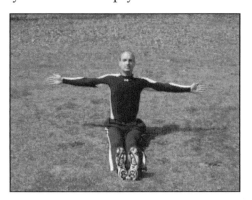
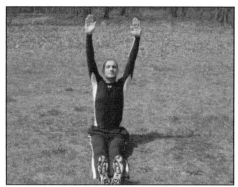

3. Close arms again causing compression to exhale completely.

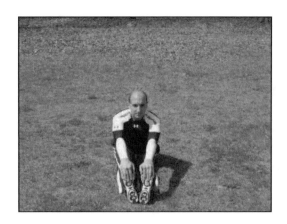

4. Repeat 8 times.

The last option, standing natural breathing, is drawn from my own personal practice and I generally include it after performing the previous three exercises. (See pictures on next page)

Standing Natural Breathing

1. Stand in a natural posture.

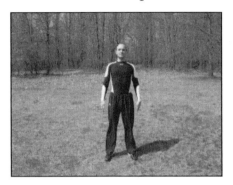 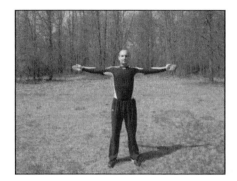

2. Stretch the arms up from the sides to above your head while inhaling.

3. Stretch a little higher.

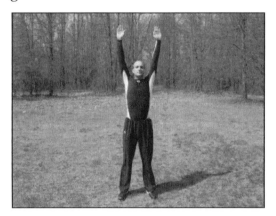

4. Exhale smoothly while simultaneously lowering your arms back down to your side. Repeat 5 to 10 times.

When performing these exercises it is important to realize that breathing is not simply a mechanical process where we see our lungs operating as a kind of bellows, drawing in and pushing out the air. Rather, we should understand that breathing is a complete physiological process of cellular respiration - our entire body breathes!

Mental imagery or visualization can aid in increasing the effectiveness of the above exercises. When inhaling, imagine the body filling up with calm, relaxing energy; feel it permeate the entire body, pouring through every cell. When exhaling, visualize all the metabolic waste products, stress, and unnecessary tensions being exhaled from the entire body. It's a very simple add-on, but it works wonderfully. Give it a try!

Keep the above exercises and principles in mind while working through the rest of this book. Breathing exercises are not meant to be done in isolation and then forgotten about during the rest of your training. I will provide suggestions for breathing patterns in the fitness exercises later on, however, please keep in mind that these are only suggestions based upon my experience. They are not dogma. Experiment with your own breathing using the principles in this section and find out what works best for you.

Leg Training for Flexibility and Power

This next set of exercises is geared towards building strength and flexibility in the legs throughout a range of motion. The ranges of motion shown here will be very familiar to Bujinkan students, yet with a slightly different spin enabling them to develop specific strength qualities necessary for their martial art. These leg exercises can be utilized for strength endurance by increasing the number of repetitions per set or, the leaping exercises can be used to develop explosive strength. Another way to do them is in a very slow, relaxed way to loosen and warm up the body for more intense training.

Jumonji Squat

1. Begin in Jumonji No Kamae (shown below) with feet slightly more than shoulder width apart.

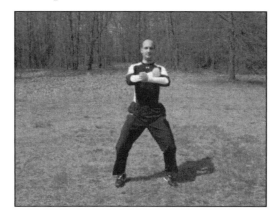

Jumonji No Kamae

2. Squat as low as possible while keeping the proper alignment of the posture.

87

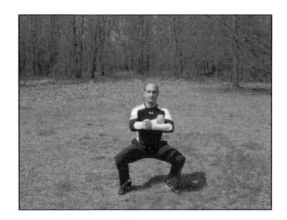

Plyometric Jumonji Jump

1. Begin in Jumonji No Kamae with feet slightly more than shoulder width apart and knees slightly bent, flexed. Legs should have a springy quality to them.

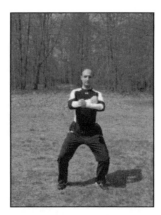

2. Leap straight up as high as possible folding the legs into the body.

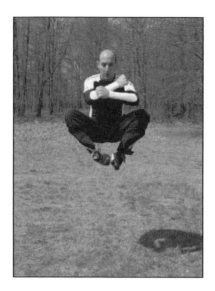

3. Land on the balls of the feet and allow the knees to bend to absorb the shock of impact. Light feet and soft knees are necessary for ninja!

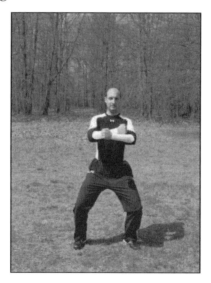

4. Immediately spring back up and continue rapidly!

Ichimonji Squat

1. Begin in a left Ichimonji No Kamae.

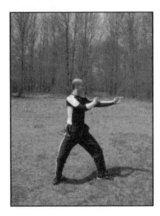

2. Squat as low as possible while keeping the proper alignment of the posture.

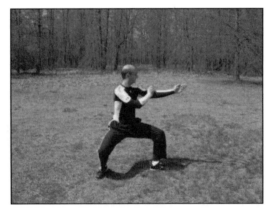

3. Switch to opposite side and continue.

Ichimonji Slow Squat

1. Begin in left Ichimonji No Kamae.
2. Begin to squat as s-l-o-w as possible while keeping the proper alignment of the posture. It should take approximately 15-20 seconds to reach the rock bottom position.

3. When you reach the bottom, pause for a few seconds before continuing upward at the same s-l-o-w pace. It should take approximately 15-20 seconds to reach top position.
4. Repeat on the other side.

Plyometric Ichimonji Jump

1. Begin in left Ichimonji No Kamae.

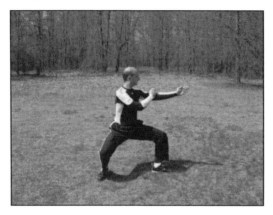

2. Leap straight up as high as possible folding the legs in to the body.

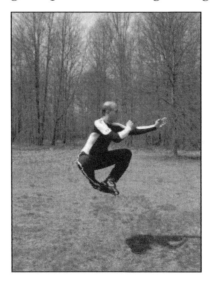

3. Land on the balls of the feet and allow the knees to bend to absorb the shock of impact. Remember to have light feet and soft knees!

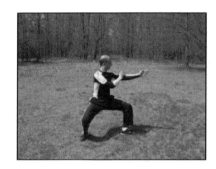

4. Immediately spring back up and continue rapidly!
5. Repeat on the opposite side.

One-legged Squat

The one legged squat, a.k.a. the "Pistol", is a great combination of strength, balance, coordination, flexibility, and muscle control.

If you are unable to do a one-legged squat the first time you attempt it, don't despair. Neither could I! This is an exercise that requires diligence, determination, and an understanding of an incremental approach to training. How do we approach this exercise incrementally? There are a few different approaches. The easiest way, in my opinion, is to hold onto something for support, i.e. – a door jam, basement pole, partner's arm, etc. This way, you are able to use as much or as little assistance as necessary to help you begin to groove the movement.

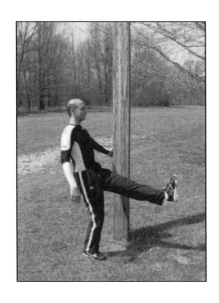 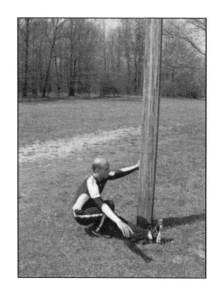

Wall Sit

This is a great isometric exercise for leg strength as well as an exercise in mental toughness. Sit against a wall, pole, tree, or even back to back with another training partner. Start with 30 seconds and try to get to 2 minutes. Another great way to use this exercise is at the end of a workout when you still feel the need to push a little bit further.

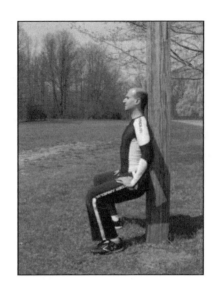

For even more of a challenge, try the Single Leg Wall Sit!

Single Leg Wall Sit

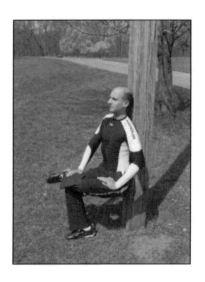

Yoko Aruki Squat

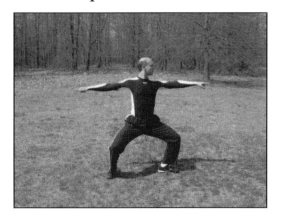 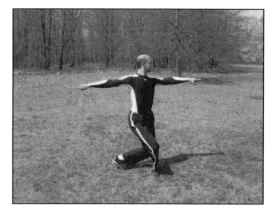

A common training principle is to greatly expand the range of motion in a particular movement (like the Yoko Aruki Squat above) in order to strengthen performance of the movement in the mid-range. In yoko aruki cross-stepping, the normal range of motion takes place within that mid-range, not the deep squat we are working on above. In addition to strengthening the mid-range of the motion, the expanded movement also is a great conditioning exercise for the legs. The complexity of this movement can be further increased by making it a plyometric movement adding in a jump. The initial step stores the elastic energy in the muscles and tendons and the subsequent release provides the required energy for the jump. In this exercise, the jump must be allowed to happen rather than forced. Don't get in your own way here!

"What is the most important ability for those who study the martial arts? It is, of course, to learn not to give up." (Hastumi, Ninpo: Wisdom for Life)

The Core of a Warrior

The core strength of the abdominal, back and gluteal muscles is the foundation from which all movement originates. Strength is the catalyst of postural endurance -- the ability to maintain core stabilization, balance and control. This is extremely relevant to Bujinkan Budo Taijutsu once we understand the implication that all movement originates from, and translates through, the core.

"The core is required to assist with respiration while also providing spinal and pelvic stabilization. These seemingly different responsibilities of the core are actually logical, harmonious functions of its design. With the proper breathing method, the mechanics and associated muscle actions of respiration will actually assist with control of intra-abdominal pressure and provide for increased stabilization of the spine and pelvic girdle." *(Internet article from Human Kinetics on Breathing)*

V-ups

1. Lie flat on your back with arms stretched out above your head.
2. Exhale, contract your core, and lift both arms and legs together to form your body into a "V" shape.
3. Inhale as you lie back down and repeat. Make sure to control this movement with appropriate core tension to avoid "flopping" back onto the ground.

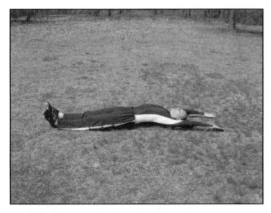

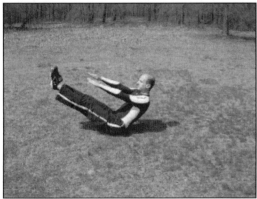

Knees to Chest

1. Begin seated with legs pulled into chest.
2. Extend legs straight out in front without your feet touching the ground.
3. Exhale, contract your core, and pull your legs back into your chest.

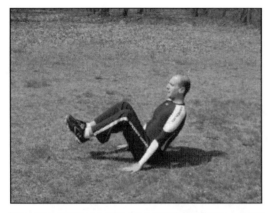

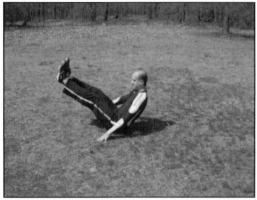

Plank

1. This can either be performed in the top portion of a push-up, or, the more difficult version, on your forearms.
2. Hold for time. Begin with 30 seconds. Continue to increase until you can hold for 5 minutes.

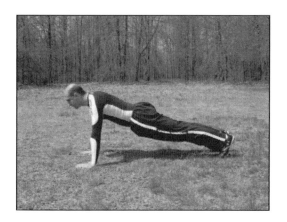 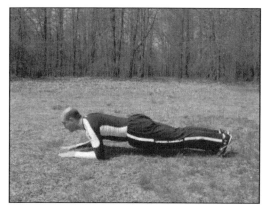

Side Plank

1. This is a great exercise to work the oblique musculature of the core.

2. Hold for time, like previous exercise.

3. Alternate sides.

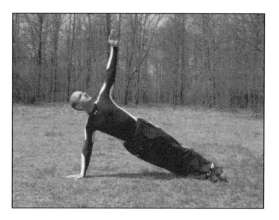

Straight Leg Sit-ups

1. Lie flat on your back.

2. Exhale, contract the core, and begin to sit up slowly keeping your spine straight.
3. Inhale at the top of the movement.
4. Exhale again and slowly lie back down.

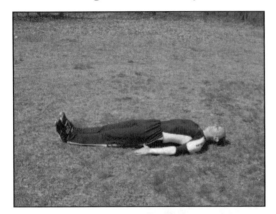
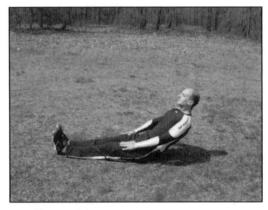
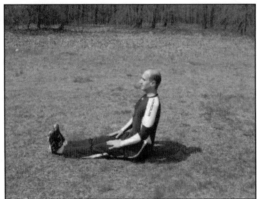

Pendulum Leg Lifts (side to side)
1. Lie on your back with your arms extended to the sides for balance.
2. Lift your feet straight up in the air.
3. Lower to the left side, but don't put them down, with legs straight
4. Bring back to center.
5. Lower to the right side and continue, side to side.

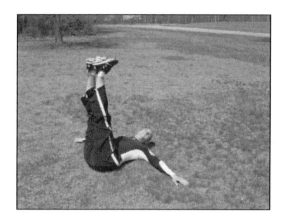
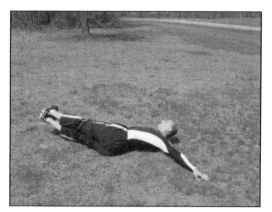
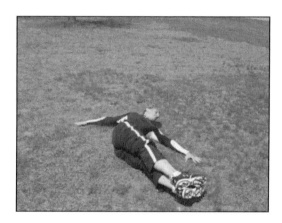

Body Drag

1. Begin in a modified Upward Facing Dog position, on your fists.
2. Exhale, contract your core, and pull your legs to your arms
3. Make sure you are not pushing with your legs – this movement should be done from the core!

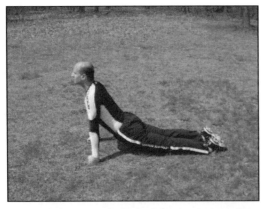

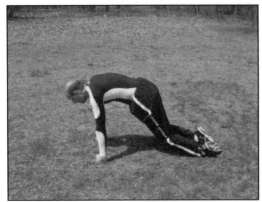

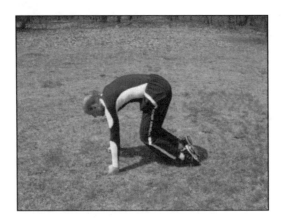

Partial Forward Roll

1. Rock back and forth to massage back muscles and spine (not shown).

Upper Body Work

Although this section is titled "upper body work", the majority of exercises presented here work the core in addition to the arms, chest, shoulders, and grip strength; nothing is worked in isolation. We work the entire body all of the time. To train like a bodybuilder (separating out different muscle groups for different days of the week) is a completely ridiculous notion for a warrior. Our training involves integrated, whole-body movement. Why would our physical fitness exercise use an opposite methodology?

Pull-ups

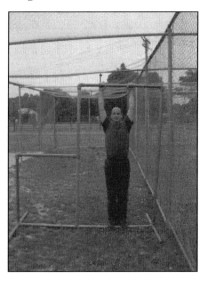 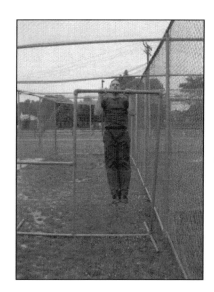

Chin-ups

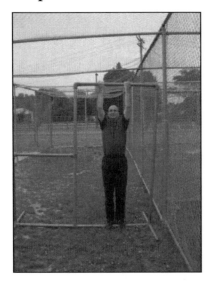 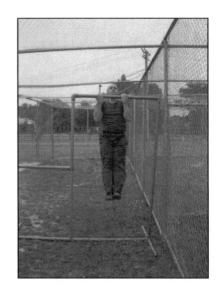

Chin-ups with L-sit

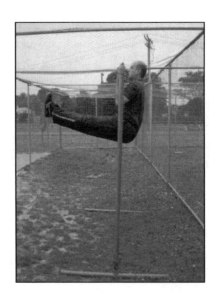

Commando Pull-ups

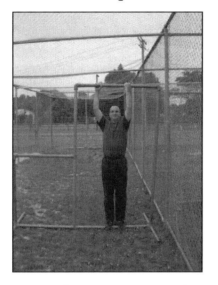 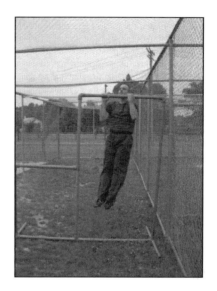

Downward Facing Dog Pushups

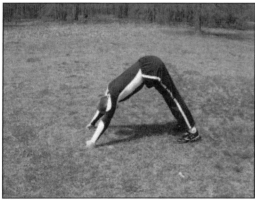 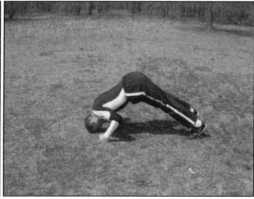

1. Begin in a downward facing dog position (these can be done with any of the various hand positions noted below).
2. Lower your head between your hands and push back up.

Hindu Push-ups

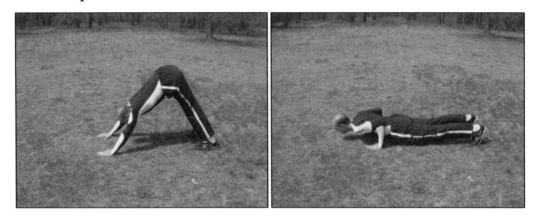

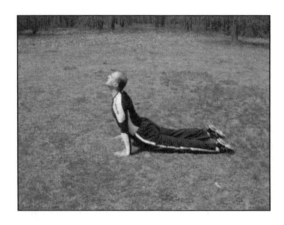

Various Fist Push-ups

These fist push-ups are used to enhance support structures for your basic strikes.

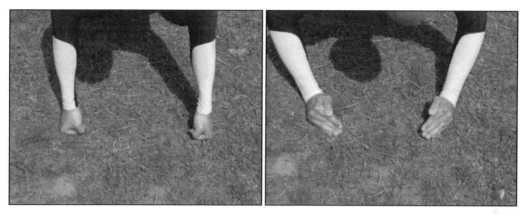

Fudo-ken

Shutou-ken

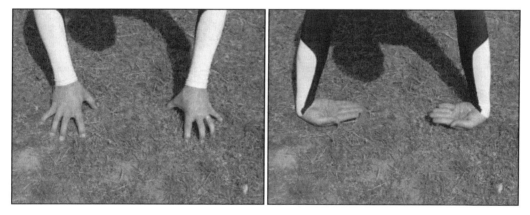

Shako-ken

Wrist push-ups

Crow Pose to Push-up

1. Squat down on the balls of your feet and place your hands on the ground in front of you.
2. Place your knees against the elbows from the outside.

3. Contract your core and tip yourself forward gently so you are balancing your entire structure on your hands.
4. Stay there for a few breaths, and then jump your legs back into a push-up position.

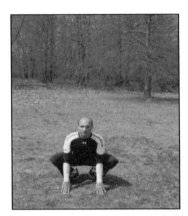 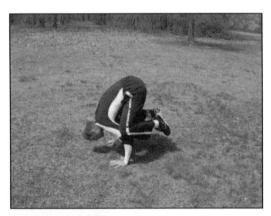

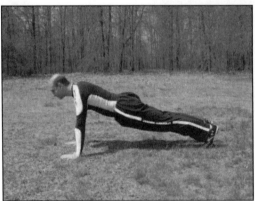

Plyometric Pushups

1. Begin as you would a regular push-up.
2. Lower down to the ground and explode up as fast as possible so that yor hands leave the ground.
3. Clap in the air before landing.
4. Continue at a furious pace!

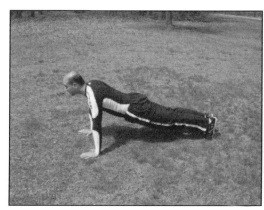
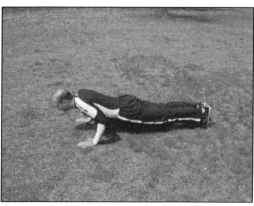
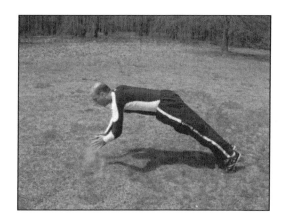

Clockwork Plyometric Pushups

1. Begin same as above in the regular Plyometric Push-up.
2. This time, as you explode upwards, your entire body leaves the ground and rotates 90 º.
3. The next push-up takes you back to center and then to the opposite side.

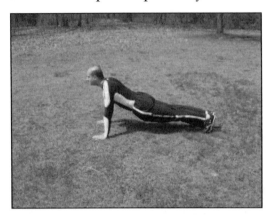
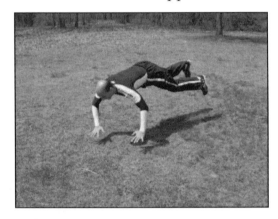
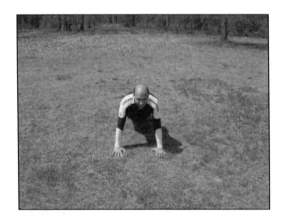

Jo Push-ups

I first saw these exercises done many years ago by an athlete using a baseball bat. The sheer creativity of them inspired me to try them, first with a hanbo, and then later with a jo. Recently, I saw a demonstration of several different variations of the same exercise on a Russian Martial Arts highlight clip online.

Seeing them being used by RMA exponents just confirmed for me the practicality and usefulness of the exercises. They will work, not only upper body strength, but core strength, coordination, and agility as well! Have fun with these!

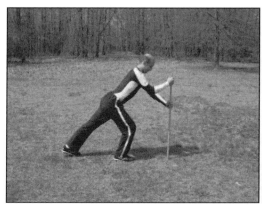
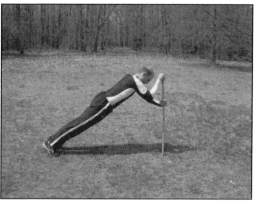
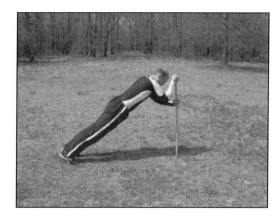

Jo Climbing

1. Begin by gripping the top of the jo, as shown below.
2. Balance the jo as you "climb" down and then back up.
3. It's harder than it looks!

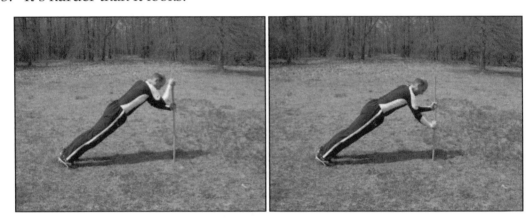

Jo Tsuki (Thrust) Push-ups

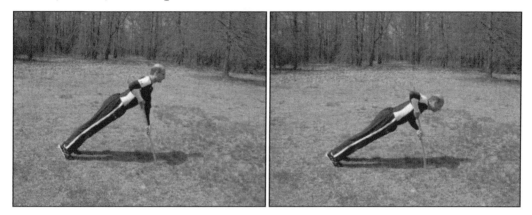

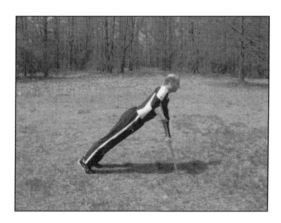

1. Balance yourself with the jo as close to vertical as possible, as if you were about to thrust.
2. Lower yourself down into the "thrust".
3. Push back to the original position.

Conditioning Exercises

Why do we need separate conditioning work added into our workout program on top of all the previous strength exercises? Simply because all the strength in the world won't do you any good if you don't have the stamina to be able to apply it when necessary. Unless you are conditioned properly, you will not be able to apply your strength or martial arts skills in a real encounter. The conditioning exercises in this section will work your entire body and help you develop that "keep going" mentality when everyone else is sitting on the sidelines.

Thoughts on "Cardio"

Many of us dedicate huge blocks of our time to "cardio" exercise in order to elevate our heart rate, increase our metabolism, and burn off extra pounds, trying to get "in-shape". But what if all that time-consuming "cardio" isn't the best way to condition yourself? What if I told you that long duration, low intensity workouts are actually a very inefficient way to lose weight and get in shape? You'd think I was nuts. Everyone knows that you must do long, exhausting "cardio" workouts to loose weight and be conditioned, right? Not exactly. Recent research has shown that the metabolic fat-burning furnace is only turned on during an aerobic workout, but turns off as soon as you stop. This means that your body is only burning fat for as long as you exercise and at a fixed rate. However, once your body adapts to the exercise you are doing, be it running on a treadmill, riding the exercise bike, fast walking, or step aerobics, the rate at which you burn fat falls off too. Not really an efficient, ideal way to lose those extra pounds now, is it?

So then what is the best way to shed those unwanted pounds? Intervals are a far better, more efficient fat-burning option that actually takes less time to perform! Intervals involve short, high intensity bursts of exercise, followed by short periods of recovery and can be used with almost any exercise (does not have to something traditionally thought of as "cardio"). An example would be to sprint all out for 30 seconds, rest for 30 seconds and repeat 8 to 10 times. This workout would take a maximum of 10 minutes, yet the metabolic furnace-stoking, fat-burning results last much longer! One research study comparing the effects of interval training versus endurance training found that the interval group lost 9 times more fat per calorie burned than the endurance group!! Impressive results.

Bear Crawls
1. Position your body so that only the palms of your hands and the balls of your feet are touching the ground.
2. Move forward, backward, left and right as fast as possible.

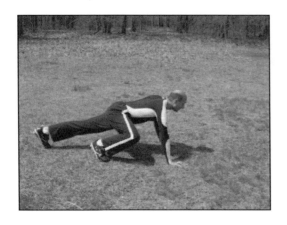
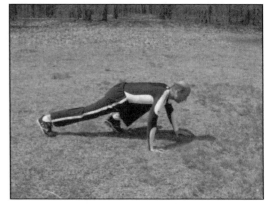

Mountain Climbers

1. From the position shown below, jump your feet back and forth as quickly as possible.

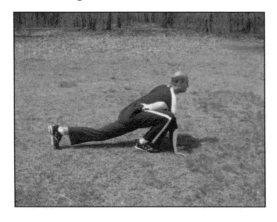
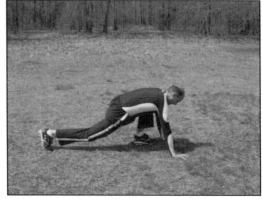

116

Stalking Tiger Push-ups

1. Begin in a pushup position with arms inverted, as shown below.
2. Now, "walk" an arm forward as you bend it.
3. Continue by moving forward, backward, and sideways, all the while performing pushups.

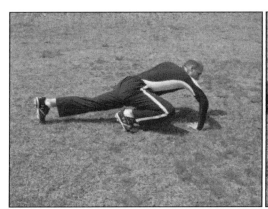 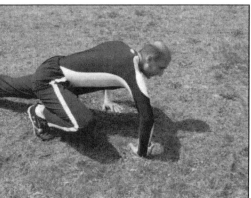

Burpees

Burpees are one of the most intense full-body conditioning exercises you can do. Enjoy them!

1. Begin in a natural stance.
2. Squat down and place both hands flat on the ground.
3. Kick your legs out to the bottom portion of a pushup position

4. Immediately jump your legs back to your hands while performing a pushup.
5. Leap up into the air and continue rapidly!

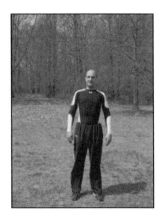
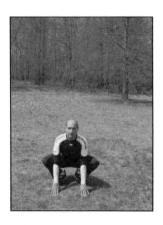
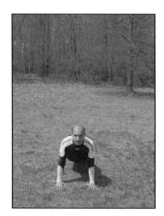
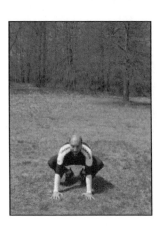
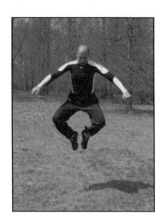

Rolling
1. From Ichimonji No Kamae, leap forward and perform a forward roll.
2. Immediately reverse direction into a back roll.

3. Leap backwards into the beginning posture.

4. Alternate sides and continue.

Happo Tenchi Tobi Nagare

1. Leap left, right, front, back, up, and down with no pause between movements. No stopping. One to the next. All 6 jumps together equal one repetition.

2. Keep jumping!

Bu-Nagare (Martial Flow)

This flow is an example of how various Warrior Fitness exercises can be combined into a sequence to train different fitness qualities together and create a synergistic type of effect. Bu-Nagare has been crafted with the intention of creating a comprehensive circuit training routine to meet the developmental needs of the aspiring Bujinkan practitioner. In the spirit of incremental progression, it is advisable to train all the components of this sequence separately at first before combining them. When you are able to perform the entire circuit in one continuous flow, one way to progress is to work through 2 rounds, rest for 60 to 90 seconds, then work through 2 more rounds. Repeat 5 times. As this becomes easier, decrease the rest period. Another idea for progression is to set a time limit, 10 or 15 minutes, and see how many rounds you can complete in the allotted time. This way, you are able to control your own rest periods; shorten, lengthen, or eliminate them as necessary.

1. Step right leg back from a natural posture into left Ichimonji No Kamae.

2. Perform two Ichimonji Squats then leap in place, switching kamae to right Ichimonji and perform two more Ichimonji Squats.

3. Jump down into the low push-up position (absorb the shock by bending the elbows and exhaling), then perform a forward roll over the left shoulder coming back into the plank (high push-up).

4. Perform an explosive Clockwork Pushup propelling the entire body counter-clockwise to the 9 o'clock position (again, remember to absorb the impact shock).

5. Lift the right arm into the air and move into Side Plank and back down to regular Plank.

6. Explosively leap back into the 12 o'clock plank position.

7. From the plank, leap up into a flat foot squat position.

8. Back roll over the left shoulder into a flat, on your stomach position.

9. Move to Upward Facing Dog back into standing right Ichimonji No Kamae. (If performing this routine underneath a pull up bar, the leap up can be to grab the bar and perform a pull up at this point before dropping back into Ichimonji No Kamae)

10. Repeat the entire sequence on the opposite side. That makes one repetition.

The incredible thing about this flow is that it combines many different aspects of fitness into one Bujinkan specific circuit routine. It simultaneously works explosive strength, strength-endurance, cardiovascular endurance, coordination, agility, and of course, mental toughness, to name several!

Concentrate on keeping proper form throughout this circuit. If you are pushing yourself too hard and the form begins to deteriorate, it's time to drop down the intensity level. You are training bad habits by pushing through the exercise without regard to form. Remember – we don't train bad habits!

Bujin Conditioning Circuit – "Pain is just weakness leaving the body."

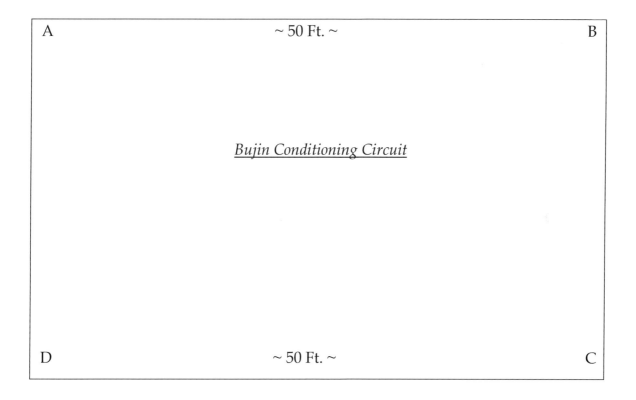

- Station "A" – 10 Burpees
- Station "B" – 10 V-ups
- Station "C" – Jo Pushups

- Station "D" – 10 Jumonji Squats

- From A to B – Sprint
- B to C – Yoko Aruki
- C to D – Bear Crawling
- D to A – Leaping

Of course this circuit is completely adaptable to all varieties of conditioning needs. Start with 5 rounds of the above circuit resting 1 to 2 minutes between rounds. As your fitness level increases, add rounds or change the temp/intensity of the exercises. The formula allows the user to plug in different exercises at each station and between stations to allow literally hundreds of permutations to ensure freshness and variety. Be creative!!

Motivation

"People often say that motivation doesn't last. Well, neither does bathing - that's why we recommend it daily."
- <u>Zig Ziglar</u>

Many people often ask me how I am able to stay motivated to train and workout on a consistent basis. The answer is pretty simple and probably surprising. Motivation is a matter of you making a daily commitment to you. You say you will do something and you do it. That's the easiest way to build trust. It's just the same as establishing trust in any relationship with another person; if you lie to them by continually breaking promises or not keeping your word, they will soon begin to doubt you and lose faith. If you lie to yourself, you will lose faith in yourself. Luckily, the converse of this statement is also true! When you keep your word to yourself by making good on your daily commitment to train and workout, you grow more confident in your belief in yourself. As you grow more confident, the commitment becomes easier and easier to keep. Start small. Make a commitment to wake up 20 minutes earlier each day for 30 days to do the head to toe joint mobility program laid out earlier in the text. Follow through on that commitment. Do it every morning for 30 days. Not only will you feel better physically throughout the day, you will begin to grow more confident in yourself because your actions truly do conform to your commitment. Don't stop there though – you're on a roll! Keep going!

"People who are unable to motivate themselves must be content with mediocrity, no matter how impressive their other talents."
- *Andrew Carnegie*

On the subject of commitment, Jack Hoban tells us at the beginning of every year how he makes the commitment to himself to go to Japan that year. The key, he says, is not asking yourself whether or not you will go (because if you approach it this way, you will never make it) but to ask yourself "how will I go?" The word "how" is important. It sends a signal to your subconscious mind telling it that it is a foregone conclusion that you ARE going; now all the mind's resources are directed to figuring out the how of going. No matter what obstacles crop up in his path, Jack's mind automatically follows the "good space" to avoid and flow around them in order to get to Japan. The very same process is also useful on a smaller scale to make a commitment to go to your weekly training classes. We all have distractions of work, family, spouses or significant others, friends, and children that serve to take us off track.

"You must train enthusiastically. When you lose enthusiasm, training becomes a problem. If you lose your enthusiasm before you are proficient at budo, your techniques will become useless [lifeless]." (Hastumi, Ninpo: Wisdom for Life)

Nike has the "just do it" slogan, but I think my brother, Dave, sums it up even more succinctly by saying, "Done!" This word has the effect of already actualizing the potential of your commitment. Get it Done.

"If you're not pushing yourself beyond the comfort zone, if you're not constantly demanding more from yourself – expanding and learning as you go – you're choosing a numb existence. You're denying yourself an extraordinary ride."
(Karnazes, Ultramarathon Man)

How Often?

How often should you train? In my opinion, you should be training every day. Everyday? Are you kidding? Jon, I have a job, I have a family, I have a life, c'mon! I can't devote every day to training! OK. Let me rephrase – every day, you should at least be doing something training related. It doesn't necessarily have to be a full-blown, high-intensity workout on daily basis because this will just lead to overtraining and injury, but at the same time, warriors are not forged by sitting on the couch watching training videos! So then, what do I mean? If you consider that every movement you make has the potential to be training then this opens up a huge array of options and new meaning to daily training. Read that again because it's a huge concept. An awareness of everyday mundane actions such as opening doors, walking to your car, sitting down, standing up, closing cabinets, taking something out of your refrigerator, etc… can all be viewed as "training" if performed with the appropriate awareness of your posture (kamae), alignment, amount of tension/force applied - are you yanking open the door to the fridge? How much force does it actually take to complete a specific action? Are you using your body (spine, hips, knees, legs) or are you isolating a particular muscle group to perform the action? When you stand up from your desk chair at work, do you hunch over, grasp the arm bars of the chair, hold your breath and force yourself up or do you smoothly lift from the crown of your head with your spine to easily and without any pause in your breathing cycle, naturally assume a standing position? This is just one small example, but it clearly illustrates my point. How you perform a particular movement is just as important, if not more important, than what you do.

"Nothing in this world can take the place of persistence. Talent will not; nothing is more common than unsuccessful men with talent. Genius will not; unrewarded genius is nearly a proverb. Education will not; the world is full of educated derelicts. Persistence and determination alone are omnipotent." – Calvin Coolidge

Creating a Training Program

Periodization is basically a fancy term for organizing and scheduling training in terms of structural units. These units are divided up into, training session, microcycle, mesocycle, macrocycle, and multiyear cycle. Periodization is a highly effective way to organize training for athletes, but what about martial artists?

There is no such thing as an off-season for a warrior. We don't need to train with the intention of "peaking" for a particular event. This being said, our training requirements are a little bit different than the average athlete, even a combat athlete. We must consistently train for multifaceted development of all-around fitness and conditioning rather than training specific strength qualities individually on a cycle-by-cycle basis. As a warrior, we need to be in a constant state of preparedness, ready for whatever real life may throw at us. Please note that a constant state of preparedness should not at all be confused with a state of hyper-vigilance. Hyper-vigilance is a psychological condition related to Post Traumatic Stress Disorder (and way beyond the scope of this book) that is highly toxic to the CNS and exhausts our physical and psychological reserves!

Below, I have put together 6 sample workout routines that cover strength endurance, explosive strength, 2 conditioning for martial arts routines, and a core work routine. They can be used separately or sown together to form a complete workout program (4 to 6 weeks), as shown in the chart below. Also, the templates can be used with all the exercises in this book to craft your own training program.

Perform 5 rounds of each circuit. Do each exercise non-stop, no pause between exercises, until you complete the round. Rest 1 to 2 minutes, then begin the next round. The volume of work can be adjusted up or down, depending on your current level of fitness. Make sure your form does not deteriorate as you begin to tire physically. If it does, ratchet down the intensity level and volume until you can perform all the exercises with good form throughout the duration.

Strength Endurance Workout

By switching up the area of the body that we are working during this circuit, we allow one area to rest and recover while movement is continuous. The benefit of this type of circuit training is that blood volume is pumped through the muscles of each working area instead of into the area (as in a typical body-building routine). This allows waste products to be carried away more efficiently and fresh blood (providing oxygen and nutrients) to be shipped in during the work.

1. Pull-ups, any variation (5)
2. Fist Push-ups (10)
3. Ichimonji Squats (10/10)
4. Hindu Push-ups (10)
5. Jumonji Squats (10)

Explosive Strength Workout

The isometric holds, followed by explosive exercises exploit what's known as the Static-Dynamic Protocol. This protocol uses the isometric holds to prime the muscles, increasing the effectiveness of the explosive exercises performed right after them.

1. Crow Pose to Push-up (10)
2. Clockwork Push-ups (10)
3. Wall Sit (1 Minute)
4. Plyometric Ichimonji Squats (10)

Conditioning for MA #1

1. Pull-ups (5)
2. Burpees (10)
3. Plyometric Jumonji Squats (10)

Conditioning for MA #2 (Minute Drills)

1. Bear Crawls (30 seconds)
2. 4 Directional Leaping – forward, backward, left, right (30 seconds)
3. Push-ups (any variation for 30 seconds)
4. Ichimonji Squats – alternating sides every 5 repetitions (30 seconds)

No rest between exercises or rounds. Move continuously through circuit 5 times for total of 10 minutes.

Core Routine

---

1. V-ups (10)
2. Pendulum Leg Raises (10)
3. Straight Leg Sit-ups (10)
4. Plank Position (1 minute hold)

Warrior Fitness Sample Training Plan

Warrior Fitness Longevity Plan		
	AM	PM
Day 1	• Joint mobility • Breathing exercises	Flow Exercises
Day 2	• Joint mobility • Breathing exercises	Conditioning Workout / Core Workout
Day 3	• Joint mobility • Breathing exercises	Martial Arts Class
Day 4	• Joint mobility • Breathing exercises	Yoga Compensatory Movement routine – 3 times through
Day 5	• Joint mobility • Breathing exercises	Strength Endurance Workout / Core Workout
Day 6	• Joint mobility • Breathing exercises	Martial Arts Class
Day 7	• Joint mobility • Breathing exercises	Explosive Strength Workout

There are numerous valid ways to design an effective workout plan that incorporates all the elements of a Warrior Fitness program. Training to develop a budo-body for warriorship must be a comprehensive endeavor. However, this does not mean that every exercise in the book should be done on a daily or even weekly basis. The routines detailed in this section, as well as the schedule above, are simply guidelines and examples of how you can tailor a program to fit your individual needs.

Please remember that any fitness exercises are supplemental to actual training and should not consume your budo training. If you only have enough time to train, then by all means train!

"Remember most of all, that the other two aspects of yourself: mind and heart, both depend on the body as their temple. Take care of your body, keep it strong, keep it ready for action." (Hoban, Ninpo: Living and Thinking as a Warrior)

Gambatte Kudasai (keep going)!!

Works Cited

Bompa, T. (1999) Periodization – Theory and Methodology of Training, 4th Edition. York University. Toronto.

Hatsumi, M. (1998) Ninpo: Wisdom for Life. Joe Maurantonio, Mushashin Press. Yonkers, NY.

Hatsumi, M. (1983) Togakure-ryu Ninpo Taijutsu. English translation by American Bujinkan Dojo. Santa Cruz, CA.

Hatsumi, M. (2004) The Way of the Ninja: Secret Techniques. Kodansha International Ltd. Bunkyo-ku, Tokyo, Japan.

Hoban, J. (1988). Ninpo: Living and Thinking as a Warrior. Contemporary Books, Inc., Chicago, IL.

Raiport, Grigori (1988). Red Gold: Peak Performance Techniques of the Russian and East German Olympic Victors. Jeremy P. Tarcher, Inc., Los Angeles, CA.

Siff, M.C. (2003). Supertraining, 6th Edition. Supertraining Institute. Denver, CO.

Verkhoshansky, Y.V. (2006) Special Strength Training – A Practical Manual for Coaches. Ultimate Athlete Concepts, Michigan, USA

About the Author

Jon Haas has been training in the Bujinkan martial arts consistently since 1989 under Shihan, senior instructor Jack Hoban. He passed the godan test in Japan during the 1999 Daikomyosai, and is currently ranked at 9th dan. For the past 12 years, Jon has been teaching a class in Mercer County Park in central NJ with his good friend and co-instructor, Josh Sager. Prior to that, Jon brought leadership to a loosely defined training group for 4 years at Fairfield University in Connecticut.

In addition to classes in Bujinkan martial arts, Jon also teaches weekly Warrior Fitness classes in the same location. For more information, please visit www.warriorfitness.org

He lives with his wife and two daughters in New Jersey.

Made in the USA
Charleston, SC
06 March 2011